LEADER'S GUIDE

THE SEVEN PILLARS *of* HEALTH

DON COLBERT, MD
with MARY COLBERT

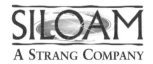

SILOAM
A STRANG COMPANY

Most STRANG COMMUNICATIONS/CHARISMA HOUSE/SILOAM/FRONTLINE/REALMS products are available at special quantity discounts for bulk purchase for sales promotions, premiums, fund-raising, and educational needs. For details, write Strang Communications/Charisma House/Siloam/FrontLine/Realms, 600 Rinehart Road, Lake Mary, Florida 32746, or telephone (407) 333-0600.

THE SEVEN PILLARS OF HEALTH LEADER'S GUIDE by Don Colbert, MD, with Mary Colbert

Published by Siloam
A Strang Company
600 Rinehart Road
Lake Mary, Florida 32746
www.siloam.com

Unless otherwise noted, all Scripture quotations are from the King James Version of the Bible.

Scripture quotations marked NIV are from the Holy Bible, New International Version. Copyright © 1973, 1978, 1984, International Bible Society. Used by permission.

Scripture quotations marked NKJV are from the New King James Version of the Bible. Copyright © 1979, 1980, 1982 by Thomas Nelson, Inc., publishers. Used by permission.

Library of Congress Control Number: 2006935330
International Standard Book Number: 978-1-59979-912-3

Neither the publisher nor the author is engaged in rendering professional advice or services to the individual reader. The ideas, procedures, and suggestions in this book are not intended as a substitute for consulting with your physician. All matters regarding your health require medical supervision. Neither the author nor the publisher shall be liable or responsible for any loss or damage allegedly arising from any information or suggestion in this book.

While the author has made every effort to provide accurate telephone numbers and Internet addresses at the time of publication, neither the publisher nor the author assumes any responsibility for errors or for changes that occur after publication.

07 08 09 10 11 — 987654321
Printed in the United States of America

PREPARING TO LEAD

Welcome to *The Seven Pillars of Health Leader's Guide! The Seven Pillars of Health* is a fifty-day program based on Dr. Don Colbert's book and includes an accompanying workbook and DVD series featuring Dr. Colbert and his wife, Mary.

This program focuses on seven key pillars that help us attain and maintain health for life through the practice of seven simple habits. The seven pillars are:

► Pillar 1: Water

► Pillar 2: Sleep and Rest

► Pillar 3: Living Food

► Pillar 4: Exercise

► Pillar 5: Detoxification

► Pillar 6: Nutritional Supplements

► Pillar 7: Coping With Stress

The Big Picture

The Seven Pillars of Health small-group program consists of a few key elements.

The Seven Pillars of Health **book.** The book is organized into fifty days of health—seven days of reading for each of the seven pillars and one final day of celebration. Dr. Colbert's teaching in this book combines sound research with years of experience. Besides discussing the modern-day environmental and societal issues that act as barriers to healthy living, Dr. Colbert also lays a solid foundation for each pillar from God's Word. Finally, the book is filled with practical tips for infusing the seven pillars of health into daily life in a natural, seamless way.

Small group sessions. The small group allows ten to twelve participants to commit to growing in divine health together through a seven-week study, plus an eighth meeting on Day 50 for a final day of celebration and reflection. In each two-hour meeting, participants watch DVD segments with Dr. Colbert and Mary, discuss what they are learning, create unique action plans for the week, and share their ongoing progress on the road toward health. Ultimately, the small group combines information, consolation, and determination to promote invigorating life change.

Daily reading. Participants commit to reading one day of *The Seven Pillars of Health* book each day and answering the corresponding questions in the workbook. On this reading schedule, they complete one pillar per week and finish the book and program in seven weeks.

Workbook and leader's guide. The workbook and leader's guide are broken into eight sessions that coincide with the seven pillars of the book plus a final day of celebration. Group members complete half of each workbook chapter during the small group meeting and the other half on their own as they read the book and answer the workbook questions during the week.

The leader's guide contains the same content as the workbook but includes all the answers to the questions. It also provides "What to Do" reminders for each activity taking place during the group meetings to help each leader lead well. The beginning of each chapter includes a Knowledge Bank, which provides a brief overview of the current pillar and key points to remember.

DVD segments. The two DVDs included in the starter kit provide the seven video segments you need to lead each meeting (pillars 1–3 on Disk 1 and pillars 4–7 on Disk 2), plus promotional materials your church can use to promote the program. Your pastor may have already invited the members of your church to participate by sharing the "Introduction to *The Seven Pillars of Health*" video clip from Disk 1 during regular Sunday services. You may also have participated in the leader training segment, found on Disk 1 under "Small Group Leader Overview," or may choose to view it prior to your first group meeting. Promotional materials, such as flyers and brochures, are available for general printing and distribution under "Support Materials" on Disk 2. (This is a DVD-ROM feature.) Please note that the DVD menu for each pillar includes a leader overview clip that better equips you for each group meeting.

Action plan. At the end of each group meeting, participants create an action plan for the upcoming week that is personalized to their own lives. This means they will commit to doing something new—a habit or simple activity—that will reinforce the knowledge they have gained for the pillar that week. The action plan commitment forms are located in the appendix of the workbook and leader's guide. After writing down their individual action plans for the week, each group member should share his or her plan with the rest of the group and then give an "action plan report" at the next meeting.

Breaking It Down

Each group meeting follows an easy format of three segments.

 HOOK UP: Let's Get Started (45 minutes)

This is a time to open the group meeting, begin with prayer, and review homework and action plans from the previous week. Five minutes have been provided for opening comments and prayer, thirty minutes for homework review, and ten minutes for action plan reports. In the first group meeting, the homework and action plan review are replaced with an icebreaker activity that allows group members to get to know one another.

 HEADS UP: Scaling the Pillars (60 minutes)

Here's where you'll find the content of each new pillar. This sixty-minute block of time begins with a short self-assessment quiz that is completely personalized and serves as a quick temperature reading for the group members' own knowledge or current habits related to that week's pillar. The group should be given about five minutes to complete the questions on their own, and then can be led quickly through a review of them by asking for a show of hands on the answers.

After the self-assessment exercise, you will share a brief overview of that week's pillar with the group. This overview information can be found in the "Give Them a Sneak Peek" section of the Knowledge Bank at the beginning of that week's chapter in the leader's guide.

Next, it's time to watch the DVD 🔘. Everyone should complete the DVD-specific questions provided in their workbooks as they watch the twenty-minute clip. Review the questions afterward with the group by asking for volunteers to share their answers.

The meeting moves into a more personal application of the week's content with a few open-ended discussion questions 👤. If you are running short on time, you do not need to cover every discussion question listed in the workbook. It's also not necessary for every group member to give an answer to every single discussion question.

Once the discussion time is over, group members need to start thinking about their action plans 🕐. A list of "thought starters" has been provided with each chapter to get the creative juices flowing, and you can review this list with the group before giving them five minutes to complete their own. Again, the action plan forms are located in the appendix. Make sure everyone shares their action plan with the rest of the group before the end of the meeting.

 TAKE IT WITH YOU: Home Study, Action, and Prayer
(15 minutes)

In this last portion of the meeting, invite group members to share any prayer requests they may have. Remind them to keep up with their action plan commitments, and give the home study assignment for the week, which is always to complete the daily reading and answer the corresponding Questions for Deeper Understanding 🐾 in the workbook each day.

Before You Lead

Make sure you have all the materials you need. On hand you should have:

- ▶ *The Seven Pillars of Health* book for each group member and yourself
- ▶ One leader's guide
- ▶ A workbook for each participant
- ▶ A complete set of DVDs
- ▶ DVD player
- ▶ Television

Before the first meeting, make sure you know who is setting up the room and the equipment. Arrive early to check that the DVD player and television are connected and that you know how to use them. Also, try previewing one of the DVDs to make sure the system is working properly. Arrange the chairs in a half-circle around the television set, and have a few extra pens and pencils on hand for the group.

We have provided a brief overview of each pillar at the beginning of each DVD for our group leaders. Review this portion of the DVD before the group convenes. (This information has also been provided in the "Give Them a Sneak Peek" section of your Knowledge Bank so that you can share an overview with the group once the meeting starts.) Also, flip through that week's portion of the book and leader's guide so that you are familiar with the material and the questions you will be asking the group.

At the first group meeting, you will want to introduce yourself, perhaps by sharing how you came to learn about the program and why you decided to lead a group. Use this time to give a brief introduction to Dr. Colbert, the seven-week program, and what they can expect from the meetings. You can read this information to the group from the "Who is Dr. Colbert?" section of your Knowledge Bank for Pillar 1.

You will also lead the group in an informal icebreaker activity at the first meeting. The instructions for this activity are listed at the beginning of Pillar 1 in this leader's guide. It's a good idea to be the first one to share in this icebreaker activity. In successive weeks, this portion of time will be devoted to homework review and updates on the previous week's action plans.

Helpful "What to Do" tips have been provided throughout the leader's guide for you. You can follow these along, and they will tell you what to do as you lead each portion of the meeting. They will also help keep the group on track and on time.

Be a Good Leader

Leading a group can seem like a daunting task, especially if it's your first time. The following tips will help ease you into this new role and help you give the best guidance you can to your group.

Be comfortable. Generally speaking, a group will be as comfortable as its leader is, especially in early sessions. Therefore, do what it takes to make yourself comfortable with the material, the room where the meetings will take place, and any equipment you will be using. Preparation is the key. Give yourself a chance to scan the week's reading and your leader's guide before the session. If possible, visit the room where the meetings will be held and be certain there are enough chairs to form a half-circle that will accommodate your group members. Check out the DVD player and learn how to start, pause, rewind, and stop it in advance. Obtain extra books in case new members join the group. This way you will feel prepared when the group meets.

Remember, you don't have to be an expert or know all the answers. Your role is to help group members to feel welcome, to lead the discussion, to keep the group on track, and to encourage group members to contribute.

Create an open atmosphere. Much of the learning will take place as group members discuss ideas learned from the book and DVDs. Therefore, it's important for the group leader to set a tone where people feel free to contribute their ideas without being "shut down" in any way. Here are some guidelines for creating an open atmosphere:

- ▶ Invite all members to contribute to the discussion without putting anyone "on the spot" to speak if they don't want to.

► Accept all contributions as worthy of consideration.

► Weave member contributions into the discussion, relating them either to something that has been said or as a starting point for the next idea.

► Make sure everyone has a chance to share. If a few talkative group members dominate the discussion, ask the group: "We've heard some good ideas from _____ and _____. What do others think?"

► Thank members for their participation and comments.

► Allow humor into the discussion.

Stay purposeful. The book and DVDs contain wonderful information for the improvement of our health. Make the most of Dr. Colbert's knowledge and research by keeping the group focused on the content of the program and moving the group from one activity to the next according to the time scheduled for each. The DVDs, workbook, and action plans are important components of the learning experience, and all activities are designed to help participants change their behaviors so they can lead healthy lives. Here are some tips for using the material in the best way for your group.

► Move quickly through the review of the self-assessment and DVD questions so that you have more time to spend on the discussion questions—these are the questions that help group members apply the material to their lives.

► Use the discussion questions as guidelines. You don't have to ask all the questions in every session. If you are running short on time, use your judgment to ask the questions that will most interest your group.

► Be sure participants have pencils/pens so they can record key points of discussion and their action plans in their workbooks.

► Never miss an opportunity to transform a comment into an idea for an action plan.

► Enlist the help of group members to track the time and give you cues when an activity should be winding up.

WEEK 1: Leading the Charge

Your Knowledge Bank for the Week

Who is Dr. Colbert, and what is The Seven Pillars of Health program?

Dr. Colbert is a board-certified medical doctor, highly trained in alternative medicine, and a Christian author and speaker with more than thirty book titles. He believes in combining alternative and traditional medical practices for optimum results in achieving optimal health. In *The Seven Pillars of Health*, he shares his life message in a program that guarantees wellness in just seven weeks.

The Seven Pillars of Health is a fifty-day program for incorporating seven basic health habits into our everyday lives: Water, Sleep and Rest, Living Food, Exercise, Detoxification, Nutritional Supplements, and Coping With Stress. The book provides seven days of reading on each pillar, which allows us to complete seven pillars in seven weeks, plus an eighth meeting on Day 50 for celebration and reflection.

Group meetings are designed to be places of information, consolation, and determination. Each meeting will include a DVD segment, followed by group discussion. Before leaving, each member will create an action plan for the week to begin introducing aspects of that week's pillar into his or her daily life. During the week, group members are responsible for daily reading and home study questions, as well as keeping up with their action plans.

Dr. Colbert's wife, Mary, joins him for lively presentations on each pillar. Group members should have *The Seven Pillars of Health* book and workbook to complete the small-group program.

Give Them a Sneak Peek: Water

Water is the single most important nutrient for our bodies and is involved in every function our bodies perform. Drinking sufficient amounts of the right kind of water can do more to improve health than anything else a person can do. It is even considered a "miracle cure"! But today, many people are not drinking adequate amounts of water and are instead replacing it with a variety of sugar-based or caffeinated drinks that do our bodies more harm than good. In addition, all water is not equal; some is safer than others.

In the DVD presentation, Dr. Colbert and Mary bring to light many of the physical ailments and symptoms that can directly result from inadequate hydration. Maladies such as joint pain and arthritis, digestion problems, headaches, dry skin, high blood pressure, allergies, weight gain, constipation, and memory loss can be helped or healed by sufficient water intake.

In the readings for Days 1–7, Dr. Colbert describes when, what kind, and how much water we should drink each day. He also outlines the "culprits" that plague our drinking water and presents the truth about modern-day water treatments, such as chlorination, fluoridation, filtration systems, and plastic packaging. Also included are guidelines for selecting and storing the best drinking water.

Key Points at a Glance

▶ Water is the single most important nutrient for our bodies and is considered a "miracle cure" for many health conditions.

▶ A body loses about two quarts of water a day through perspiration, urination, and exhalation.

▶ Waiting until we are thirsty to drink water most likely means we are already dehydrated.

▶ Many symptoms of disease are the same indicators our bodies give when they need a more adequate intake of water.

▶ Water slows the aging process and helps maintain brain function.

▶ Water straight from a faucet may contain toxins, heavy metals, pesticides, bacteria, and other microbes.

▶ Of the two types of fluoride—sodium fluoride, which is added to toothpaste, and sodium silicofluoride, which is added to drinking water—the latter is more harmful.

▶ Some bottled waters contain more toxins than tap water and are not as closely regulated as tap water.

▶ Distilled water and water filtered by reverse osmosis are the purest to drink because they've been stripped of all foreign substances. However, because they are also stripped of any minerals, they become highly acidic once in our bodies.

▶ Alkaline water filters are the best type of filters because our bodies thrive best in an alkaline environment.

PILLAR 1: Water

And the earth was without form, and void; and darkness was upon the face of the deep. And the spirit of God moved upon the face of the waters.

—GENESIS 1:2

Jesus answered and said unto her, Whosoever drinketh of this water shall thirst again: But whosoever drinketh of the water that I shall give him shall never thirst; but the water that I shall give him shall be in him a well of water springing up into everlasting life.

—JOHN 4:13–14

 HOOK UP: Let's Get Started (45 minutes)

Welcome (10 minutes)

WHAT TO DO

Welcome the group members and introduce the program by reading the "Who is Dr. Colbert?" section in your Knowledge Bank.

Open with prayer (5 minutes)

Icebreaker (30 minutes)

WHAT TO DO

Lead the group in an icebreaker activity by asking everyone to introduce themselves by sharing:
- ▶ Their name
- ▶ One item from their pocket, purse, or wallet that tells something about them
- ▶ Why they joined this study

Be the first to introduce yourself with a personal object.

HEADS UP: Scaling the First Pillar (60 minutes)

WHAT TO DO

Give the group five minutes to complete the following self-assessment quiz. Review answers with a show of hands.

---

1. How many ounces of water would you say you drank yesterday?

    ☐ Eight ounces or less

    ☐ Sixteen ounces

    ☐ Thirty-two ounces

    ☐ Sixty-four ounces or more

    ☐ Don't know

2. From what source do you get your drinking water?

    ☐ Tap

    ☐ Plastic bottle

    ☐ Glass bottle

    ☐ Drinking fountain

    ☐ Water filtration system (i.e., reverse osmosis, carbon filter)

3. What other drinks did you consume yesterday? List the amounts in ounces (it's OK to estimate):

Drink	Amount in ounces
Coffee	
Tea	
Soft drink	
Fruit juice	
Sugar-based "juice" drink	
Alcoholic beverage	
Other: _____	

4. When do you tend to drink water?

    ☐ Morning

    ☐ Afternoon

    ☐ Evening

    ☐ During meals

    ☐ Whenever I am thirsty

5. About how much water do you believe you should drink every day?

    ☐ Sixteen ounces

    ☐ Thirty-two ounces

    ☐ Sixty-four ounces

    ☐ As much as my body tells me to

6. Where do you believe the healthiest water comes from?

    ☐ Tap water

    ☐ Spring water

    ☐ Bottled water

    ☐ Distilled water

    ☐ Filtered water

BE IN THE KNOW

Our bodies thrive in an alkaline environment. When we are properly alkalinized, our tissues rid themselves of impurities quickly and detoxify themselves much more efficiently. To boost your body from its acidic environment toward a robust, healthy alkaline level instead, drink bottled alkalinized water or install an alkalizing filter in your home.

LISTEN UP: Learning From the Expert

WHAT TO DO

Before playing the DVD, share some "Sneak Peek" information from your Knowledge Bank with the group. Start the DVD, and tell the group to answer the DVD questions as they watch. After the video, ask for volunteers to answer each question.

Name some specific body parts and processes that depend on water for proper functioning.

Our blood, lymphatic fluid, immune system, digestive and respiratory tracts, joints and disks, brain, spine, eyes, muscles, and brain cells require water in order to function properly.

What are a few of the reasons we should avoid drinking tap water?

The environment has made groundwater unhealthy. New chemicals get assimilated into our groundwater. Chlorine and fluoride are often added to tap water in the filtration process.

What is the formula for determining how much water to drink each day?

Take our body weight, divide it by two, and aim to drink that many ounces in water daily.

 SPEAK UP: Let's Talk About It

WHAT TO DO

Discussion questions are meant to promote interaction with the material on a personal level. Ask people to share their responses if they feel comfortable.

What *aha!* moment did you have while listening to Dr. Colbert's message?

Answers will vary.

What point does Dr. Colbert make that is especially relevant to your own life and health habits right now?

Answers will vary.

Given the Scripture verses shared by the Colberts on the DVD and provided at the beginning of this chapter, how is this pillar relevant to our faith?

Answers will vary.

Additional notes:

_____

_____

_____

 PUT IT ALL IN MOTION: Creating an Action Plan

WHAT TO DO

Explain that an action plan is a formal commitment to do something different during the week as a result of what we have learned. The action plans are located in the appendix (page 76 in the workbook and page 101 in the leader's guide). Review the thought starters provided here to help spark some creative ideas. Then give the group five minutes to write their individual action plans for the week. Afterward, ask each person to share their plan with the group.

THOUGHT STARTERS FOR YOUR ACTION PLAN

- ▶ In light of what the self-assessment you completed at the beginning of our study revealed, how will you change your drinking habits this week?
- ▶ What research might you do to find out more about the water you drink?
- ▶ Is it time to change the brand of water you currently drink? How about installing a water filter in your home?
- ▶ Keep a journal of how much water you drink and what time of day you drink it.

TAKE IT WITH YOU: Home Study, Action, and Prayer
(15 minutes)

WHAT TO DO

Take prayer requests from the group. Share the home study assignment listed below, and remind everyone to keep up with their action plans—they will give a report on how they did at the next meeting. To finish the meeting, ask someone to close in prayer.

List prayer requests for this week here. Remember to pray for one another this week.

_____

_____

_____

_____

Close in prayer.

Keep up with this week's action plan.

Home study assignment: Read Days 1–7 in *The Seven Pillars of Health* and answer the Questions for Deeper Understanding on the following pages.

 Questions for Deeper Understanding Days 1–7

DAY 1 — — — — — — — — — — — —

Why does Dr. Colbert refer to water as a miracle cure?

> *Because most of the physical ailments plaguing people can be "cured" through a greater intake of water each day. Most people are living in a mildly dehydrated state and treating the corresponding symptoms with Tylenol, Advil, Prozac, and many other prescription drugs—but what their bodies really need is an adequate intake of water every day.*

What physical ailment or discomfort of yours might be alleviated with greater water intake?

Answers will vary.

DAY 2 — — — — — — — — — — — —

What are the "starting five" of the vital organs?

The brain, heart, lungs, liver, and kidneys.

List a few health conditions and how they are complicated by dehydration.

Joint pain and arthritis—if our cartilage is robbed of fluid, the joints eventually creak, crack, and pop. Over an extended period of time, this degenerative process may lead to arthritis.

High blood pressure—dehydration restricts the flow of blood to some areas of the body, concentrating instead on the most vital organs, and may lead to high blood pressure.

Digestion problems—because water is the basis of every fluid our bodies need for the digestive process, the whole digestive system goes into emergency mode without enough water. The result? Heartburn, indigestion, constipation, hemorrhoids, and even ulcers may occur.

Asthma—a higher histamine level, which results from inadequate hydration, causes the muscles in the bronchial tubes to constrict, thus restricting the flow of air.

DAY 3 — — — — — — — — — — — —

How does water act as an unending fountain of youth?

Water rejuvenates our skin, making us look years younger and keeping the skin hydrated and elastic. It also keeps our memory sharp, even as we age, and helps us lose weight and feel great.

In what areas would you like to see water help improve your appearance?

Answers will vary.

DAY 4 — — — — — — — — — — — — —

Why is there more concern about the water we drink today than in past years?

> With the advent of the Industrial Revolution, our environment is plagued with the adverse effects of smokestacks, plastics, and agri-pollution. Since whatever goes into the environment eventually settles into our natural sources of water, our drinking water is now infected with many contaminants and toxins.

What specific contaminants threaten our water now?

> Carcinogens, pesticides, herbicides, fertilizers, pharmaceutical products, parasites, chlorine, fluoride, and aluminum.

What health risks do they pose?

> We can be plagued with giardia, intestinal flu, miscarriages, birth defects, osteosarcoma, calcium deposits, arthritis, and the disruption of vitamin and mineral functions.

DAY 5 — — — — — — — — — — — — —

Is bottled water always a good choice? Why or why not?

> It depends on the source. Some bottled waters are no better than tap water in fancy packaging!

Why shouldn't we reuse water bottles?

> Dangerous bacteria can accumulate in and on the plastic as it is reused.

What guidelines will help you select the safest bottled water?

> Check to see if the manufacturer is a member of IBWA. Choose glass bottles over plastic ones. Drink water within a few months of its bottling date. Check the mineral content.

DAY 6 — — — — — — — — — — — —

Describe the difference between an alkaline and an acidic environment in the body.

An alkaline environment rids our tissues of impurities more quickly, while an acidic environment is less efficient at removing toxins.

How can you promote a greater alkaline environment in your body?

Drink alkaline waters and eat alkaline foods. Test your urine pH level. Purchase an alkalizing filter for your home.

Use the chart below to describe the benefits and limitations of the different water filtration systems.

TYPE OF FILTRATION	PROS	CONS
Carbon—granulated	*Inexpensive; removes chlorine and most lead*	*Doesn't filter out many toxins*
Carbon—block	*Lasts longer and filters microorganisms better than granulated carbon filters*	*Costs more than a granulated carbon filter; doesn't remove fluoride, viruses, or other tap water impurities very effectively*
Distillation	*Removes every impurity, including chloride, fluoride, bacteria, parasites, and heavy metals*	*Removes good minerals, too, and may make our bodies acidic*
Reverse osmosis	*Removes every impurity*	*More expensive than other filters; may make our bodies acidic*
Alkaline	*Converts filtered water to alkaline water*	*Must use water that is rich in minerals, not water that is distilled or has been filtered through reverse osmosis*

DAY 7 — — — — — — — — — — — —

Based on Dr. Colbert's formula, how many ounces of water should you be drinking each day?

> *Answers will vary. The formula is to take one-half your body weight and drink that many ounces a day.*

When are the best times of day to drink water?

> *Thirty minutes before a meal, two hours after a meal, and before 7:00 p.m.*

What foods will increase your water intake?

> *Salads, tomatoes, lettuce, vegetables, bananas, apples, and watermelon. In other words, all fruits and veggies!*

WEEK 2: Leading the Charge

Your Knowledge Bank for the Week

Give Them a Sneak Peek: Sleep and Rest

Dr. Colbert likens the value of a good night's sleep to the vital cleanup operation that occurs every night at Walt Disney World. If thorough cleanups don't happen, the whole theme park starts to run down and, ultimately, loses its luster and appeal.

So too with our physical bodies. During sleep, our bodies shut down and repair themselves, replacing old cells with new ones and recharging the immune system. Simply put, the sleep restores us to optimum health and vitality.

In the DVD presentation, Dr. Colbert and Mary talk about the importance of getting seven to nine hours of sleep each night. Adequate sleep means improved brain function, a boost to the immune system, slowed aging, resistance to disease, and more. Fortunately, many "enemies" of sleep—such as too much caffeine, anxiety, painful physical conditions, and eating the wrong foods—have practical antidotes.

The readings for Days 8–14 detail those antidotes, which range from getting plenty of exercise to corralling our thoughts, from focusing on what we're thankful for to planning ahead for a good night's sleep, and from maintaining a relaxing sleep environment to eating the right foods. Dr. Colbert outlines acceptable sleep aids and provides a chart for keeping track of sleep habits to better understand sleep patterns. He also encourages readers to create an appreciation list to help ease their anxiety and promote peacefulness and rest.

Key Points at a Glance

- A good night's sleep repairs, restores, and rejuvenates the body.

- Sleep cares for the immune system, slows the aging process, and deters the development of type 2 diabetes and other diseases.

- Insomnia robs people of sleep and, in the long run, good health. Stress, anxiety, depression, chronic pain, caffeine, and medications all contribute to the onset of insomnia.

- Sugary or highly processed foods may produce low blood sugar levels, which can make sleep difficult.

- ► Stages three and four of the regular sleep cycle are the most restful and important for our bodies.

- ► Dreams help restore the mind.

- ► Nightly bedtime rituals help establish a good night's sleep.

- ► Exercise improves the quality of our sleep.

- ► Snoring may be a sign of sleep apnea.

- ► Take time to relax before bedtime.

- ► To create a sleep-conducive environment, keep the bedroom dark, filter out noises, secure a good mattress and pillow, and set the temperature to a comfortable level.

- ► Instead of relying on over-the-counter or prescribed sleep medications, try more natural and healthier sleep aids, such as valerian, 5-HTP, L-theanine, bedtime teas, or other sources of calcium, melatonin, and magnesium.

- ► Days of rest are one of the most basic principles of good health.

PILLAR 2: Sleep and Rest

He grants sleep to those he loves.

—Psalm 127:2, niv

Come to me, all you who are weary and burdened, and I will give you rest.

—Matthew 11:28, niv

Thou wilt keep him in perfect peace, whose mind is stayed on thee: because he trusteth in thee.

—Isaiah 26:3

 HOOK UP: Let's Get Started (45 minutes)

Welcome; open with prayer (5 minutes)

Health checkup: homework review (30 minutes)

Action plan progress report (10 minutes)

WHAT TO DO

Welcome everyone back to the group and open the time with a short prayer. Then review the homework questions from last week. Invite volunteers to share answers as they feel comfortable. After the homework review, ask each group member to remind everyone of their action plan from the previous week and share how they did in keeping up with it.

 HEADS UP: Scaling the Second Pillar (60 minutes)

WHAT TO DO

Give the group five minutes to complete their self-assessment quiz. Review answers with a show of hands.

---

1. How much sleep do you get on a normal night?

    ▢ Less than six hours

    ▢ Six to seven hours

    ▢ Eight hours or more

2. Do you feel refreshed in the morning?

    ▢ Always

    ▢ Sometimes

    ▢ Never

3. What time do you normally fall asleep?

    ▢ Before 10:00 p.m.

    ▢ Between 10:00 and 11:00 p.m.

    ▢ Between 11:00 p.m. and midnight

    ▢ After midnight

4. If you wake up in the middle of the night and have trouble falling back to sleep, what do you do to fall asleep again?

    ▢ Read a book

    ▢ Watch TV

    ▢ Wake up my partner

    ▢ Go to the kitchen to grab a late-night snack

    ▢ Lie in bed thinking about what I did today or planning about tomorrow

5. How long does it take you to fall asleep?

    ▢ Fifteen minutes

    ▢ Fifteen to thirty minutes

    ▢ More than thirty minutes

6. Which, if any, of the following sleep aids do you use?

    ▢ Sleep-Eze

    ▢ Tylenol PM

Herbal tea drink

    I don't use anything.

7. Which of the following items are in your bedroom right now?

    Sewing machine

    Office equipment (computer, fax machine)

    Clean laundry

    Exercise equipment

 LISTEN UP: Learning From the Expert

WHAT TO DO

Before playing the DVD, share some "Sneak Peek" information from your Knowledge Bank with the group. Start the DVD, and tell the group to answer the DVD questions as they watch. After the video, ask for volunteers to answer each question.

Why did God command the Sabbath?

> *He created our bodies to need rest regularly. Ultimately, He commanded it because He knew we would need it.*

What work does our body accomplish while we sleep?

> *Sleep regulates the release of important hormones, like growth hormone or leptin. It recharges the body, helps prevent cancer, improves brain function and memory, reduces stress, and helps energize us.*

Why is the term "beauty rest" such an apt phrase?

> *Adequate sleep slows the aging process.*

Name some dangers of inadequate sleep.

> *Increased risk of type 2 diabetes, slowed reaction time, shorter attention span, impaired memory and coordination, impaired decision-making ability, higher stress, reduced workplace productivity, other lives endangered on the road, jeopardized marriage, and disease*

BE IN THE KNOW

Are you sleep deprived? Try sitting in a comfortable chair in a quiet, darkened room for five minutes. If you fall asleep, you are certainly deprived of the sleep your body needs.

 SPEAK UP: Let's Talk About It

WHAT TO DO

Discussion questions are meant to promote interaction with the material on a personal level. Ask people to share their responses if they feel comfortable.

How important a role have sleep and rest played in your life lately?

Answers will vary.

What factors are hindering you from getting adequate sleep and rest?

Answers will vary.

What adverse effects, if any, have resulted from a lack of sleep and rest in your life?

Answers will vary.

Given the Scripture verses shared by the Colberts on the DVD and provided at the beginning of this chapter, how is this pillar relevant to our faith?

Answers will vary.

Additional notes:

_____

_____

_____

PUT IT ALL IN MOTION: Creating an Action Plan

WHAT TO DO

Review the thought starters provided here to help spark some creative ideas for this week's action plans. The action plans are located in the appendix (page 76 in the workbook and page 101 in the leader's guide). Give the group five minutes to write their plan for the week. Afterward, ask each person to share theirs with the group.

THOUGHT STARTERS FOR YOUR ACTION PLAN

- ▶ Keep a sleep journal for seven days, recording time to bed, hours of sleep, how you felt when you woke up, and factors that may have contributed to a good or bad night's sleep. See page 48 in *The Seven Pillars of Health* for a sample journal page.
- ▶ How can you make your bedroom environment more relaxing and conducive to sleep?
- ▶ Will you abstain from certain foods, drinks, habits, or medications before bedtime?
- ▶ Purchase soft earplugs or a sound generator to block noises while you sleep.

 TAKE IT WITH YOU: Home Study, Action, and Prayer
(15 minutes)

WHAT TO DO

Take prayer requests from the group. Share the home study assignment listed below, and remind everyone to keep up with their action plans—they will give a report on how they did at the next meeting. To finish the meeting, ask someone to close in prayer.

List prayer requests for this week here. Remember to pray for one another this week.

_____

_____

_____

_____

Close in prayer.

Keep up with this week's action plan.

Home study assignment: Read Days 8–14 in *The Seven Pillars of Health* and answer the Questions for Deeper Understanding on the following pages.

 Questions for Deeper Understanding Days 8–14

DAY 8 — — — — — — — — — — — — — — —

Name some ways that sleep and rest improve your health.

> *Sleep regulates the release of important hormones, slows the aging process, boosts the immune system, improves brain function, and reduces cortisol levels.*

How has sleep deprivation affected your work performance at some point in your life?

> *Answers will vary.*

DAY 9 — — — — — — — — — — — — — — —

Which "sleep thieves" have been robbing you of sleep? Check all that apply to you.

> *Answers will vary.*

☐ Stress, anxiety, or depression   ☐ Alcohol

☐ Painful physical conditions   ☐ Exercise

☐ Newborn baby   ☐ Snoring spouse

☐ Low-carb diet   ☐ Hot flashes/menstrual cramps

☐ Food insomnia   ☐ Bad mattress or pillow

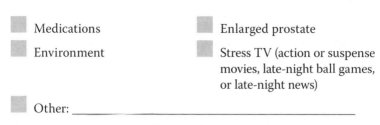

☐ Medications

☐ Environment

☐ Enlarged prostate

☐ Stress TV (action or suspense movies, late-night ball games, or late-night news)

☐ Other: _____

Are these statements true or false? If false, correct the statement so that it becomes true.

☑ T ☐ F   Caffeine remains in the body up to twenty hours.

☑ T ☐ F   Instant coffee is less caffeinated than brewed coffee.

☑ T ☐ F   Some over-the-counter headache remedies contain caffeine.

☑ T ☐ F   Too much protein increases the need for more sleep.

☐ T ☑ F   Green tea contains antioxidants but no caffeine.

Eight ounces of green tea contains 30 mg of caffeine.

Name some drinks, medicines, or foods you want to avoid near bedtime.

Caffeinated drinks, alcohol, decongestants, some pain relievers, certain antidepressants, blood pressure and thyroid medications, prednisone, hormone replacements, and foods high in sugar or highly processed, like ice cream, cake, and popcorn.

DAY 10 — — — — — — — — — — — —

What lifestyle adjustments can you make to reach the goal of seven to nine hours of sleep each night?

Answers will vary.

Reflect on a dream you had recently. What happened? How did you feel afterward? What circumstances in your life may have contributed to your having had that dream?

Answers will vary.

How have you regarded your dreams in the past—relevant and revealing, or disturbing and a nuisance? Are you inclined to accept Dr. Colbert's perspective that they help us reflect on serious issues in our lives?

Answers will vary.

DAY 11 — — — — — — — — — — — — — —

What bedtime snacks do you normally consume?

> *Answers will vary.*

Which of Dr. Colbert's approved bedtime snacks are you inclined to choose instead?

> *Answers will vary.*

How might using an appreciation list help improve your sleep and rest?

> *Many times our sleep suffers because we dwell on potential problems or past failures. An appreciation list helps convert those worries into praises, which then promotes peace and restfulness.*

DAY 12 — — — — — — — — — — — — — —

Which of the tips Dr. Colbert gives for "planning" a good night's sleep from Days 11 and 12 have you already incorporated into your lifestyle?

> *Answers will vary.*

- Exercise during the day.
- Get rid of clutter in the bedroom.
- Dim the lights in the living areas before bedtime.
- Eliminate light in the bedroom such as clocks, nightlights, etc.
- Play soft music near bedtime.
- Eliminate light coming into the bedroom from outside sources by lining the drapes or pulling down a dark shade.
- Take a warm bath or shower before bed.
- Click off the "worry channel" in your mind.
- Have a light snack balanced with protein, carbohydrates, and fats.
- Avoid the news or violent programs.
- Use a sound generator to produce "white noise."
- Use earplugs.
- Use Breathe Right strips or Snore Eze.

☐ Set the room temperature at a more comfortable setting.

☐ Other: _____

Of those listed that you currently do not do, which will you incorporate, and how do you think they will help?

Answers will vary.

If your mattress is too hard or too soft, are you willing to invest in a new one? What commitments would such an investment require from you?

Answers will vary.

DAY 13 — — — — — — — — — — — —

On the following chart, draw a line from the acceptable sleep aid in the left-hand column with its appropriate characteristic on the right. One answer is given for you.

Valerian	Decreases the time it takes to fall asleep and does not cause daytime drowsiness
5-HTP	A hormone that may be missing in people advanced in age
Calcium	Low levels can lead to fatigue, confusion, irritability, weakness, muscle cramps, and insomnia
Magnesium	Very effective at raising levels of serotonin, which helps alleviate symptoms of stress, anxiety, and depression while improving sleep
L-theanine	Important in the contraction of muscles and the release of neurotransmitters that can support sleep
Melatonin	Found naturally in the green tea plant; promotes relaxation, calms nervousness, and decreases restlessness
Bedtime teas	Soothing to drink one or two hours before bed

What has your sleep journal been revealing about your sleep habits?

Answers will vary.

DAY 14

What activities do you enjoy that promote restfulness for your mind, body, and spirit?

Answers will vary.

How can you allocate time in your weekly schedule for restful activities such as these?

Answers will vary.

WEEK 3: Leading the Charge

Your Knowledge Bank for the Week

Give Them a Sneak Peek: Living Food

The reading for this week opens with a challenge: survey your pantry, refrigerator, and freezer to make note of the kinds of food you buy, store, and eat. Are they living foods or dead foods?

Just as the terms denote, living foods contribute to our health, while dead foods breed disease. Unfortunately, the "standard American diet" of fast-food convenience is high in refined sugars and dangerous fats—all dead foods. Dr. Colbert and Mary discuss the impact of poor food choices, which we have often inherited from our parents, on our health. They tout the benefits of living foods, attractively packaged in skins and peels, over dead foods that have been enhanced and encased in careful packaging to ensnare and addict us.

In the readings for Days 15–21, Dr. Colbert details which foods to eat and which foods to avoid. He offers healthful rules of thumb for choosing and cooking vegetables, meats, seafood, dairy products, and fats. He explains the harmful effects of sugar, white flour, and fried foods, and he instructs us on the bad fats to avoid. This pillar includes charts that help us with food selection, such as a glycemic index for fruits and vegetables and lists of calcium-rich foods, recommended fish, and the best and worst cooking oils. It also includes a body mass index and a formal "Agreement to Lose Weight" that readers can sign in their resolve to practice more healthful eating habits.

Key Points at a Glance

▶ Everything we put in our mouth has the potential to produce life or death.

▶ Living foods are packaged in divinely created wrappers called skins and peels; they are prepared by being plucked, harvested, or squeezed.

▶ Dead foods have been altered through harmful cooking processes or the addition of preservatives, chemicals, hormones, or other additives.

▶ Fruits, vegetables, whole grains, and healthy oils are all living foods.

▶ God originally designed man to be a vegetarian.

- The more processed a food is, the more sugar it contains and the more harm it will do to the body, especially if it contains hydrogenated or partially hydrogenated fats.

- Limit the intake of fatty meats, such as bacon, sausage, hot dogs, and cold cuts.

- Not all fats are bad. Good alternatives are extra-virgin olive oil, almonds, macadamia nuts, and flaxseeds.

- Choose whole-grain breads, pastas, and cereals.

- Consume five to thirteen servings of fruits and vegetables a day.

- When choosing meats, choose the leanest cuts of free-range or grass-fed meats, and avoid those that have been irradiated.

- Wild Alaskan salmon, halibut, sardines, tilapia, and sole are the best fish for you. They contain less mercury than most other fish and are sources of omega-3 fatty acids.

- Dark chocolate is high in antioxidants and can be good for you in small amounts.

- Avoid aluminum and Teflon-coated cookware. Cook foods in CorningWare, glassware, or stainless steel cookware instead.

- Eating food too quickly sends wrong messages to your body. Chew each bite twenty to thirty times.

PILLAR 3: Living Food

"Everything is permissible for me"—but not everything is beneficial. "Everything is permissible for me"—but I will not be mastered by anything.

—1 CORINTHIANS 6:12, NIV

Jesus said to them, "My food is to do the will of Him who sent Me, and to finish His work."

—JOHN 4:34, NKJV

Do you not know that your body is the temple of the Holy Spirit who is in you, whom you have from God, and you are not your own? For you were bought at a price; therefore glorify God in your body and in your spirit, which are God's.

—1 CORINTHIANS 6:19–20

 HOOK UP: Let's Get Started (45 minutes)

Welcome; open with prayer (5 minutes)

Health checkup: homework review (30 minutes)

Action plan progress report (10 minutes)

WHAT TO DO

Welcome everyone back to the group and open the time with a short prayer. Then review the homework questions from last week. Invite volunteers to share answers as they feel comfortable. After the homework review, ask each group member to remind everyone of their action plan from the previous week and share how they did in keeping up with it.

HEADS UP: Scaling the Third Pillar (60 minutes)

WHAT TO DO

Give the group five minutes to complete their self-assessment quiz. This self-assessment covers information that actually has right or wrong answers, and the answers have been provided for you. After asking for volunteers to answer the questions, feel free to share the correct answers with the group.

1. According to the U.S. Department of Agriculture (USDA) dietary guidelines, about how many servings of fruits and vegetables do you think the average person should eat daily?

    ☐ Two to three

    ☐ Four to ten

    ✔ Five to thirteen

    ☐ Eight to ten

2. "Bad" fats include (check all the right answers):

    ☐ Monounsaturated fats

    ☐ Omega-3 fatty acids

    ✔ Hydrogenated fats

    ✔ Saturated fats (excessive amounts)

3. Which of the oils listed below are the healthiest?

    ✔ Olive oil

    ✔ Flaxseed oil

    ✔ Fish oil

    ☐ Corn oil

    ☐ Safflower oil

BE IN THE KNOW

Food companies know exactly what they are doing. Not only do they hire savvy marketers and psychologists to package their processed foods in a way they're certain will appeal to you, but they also hire the brightest minds and chemists to create dead foods that have eye appeal and the tastes, textures, feels, and smells that will make them as addictive and irresistible to you as possible.

4. Which of the nuts listed here are healthiest?

    ☐ Peanuts

    ☐ Cashews

    ✓ Almonds

    ✓ Walnuts

    ✓ Macadamia

5. Which sweet is considered healthy?

    ☐ M&Ms

    ☐ Oreo cookies

    ☐ Snickers candy bar

    ✓ Dark chocolate

 LISTEN UP: Learning From the Expert

WHAT TO DO

Before playing the DVD, share some "Sneak Peek" information from your Knowledge Bank with the group. Start the DVD, and tell the group to answer the DVD questions as they watch. After the video, ask for volunteers to answer each question.

What is the difference between getting a cold or the flu and getting cancer, heart disease, or diabetes?

> *We catch a cold or the flu, but we develop cancer, heart disease, and diabetes.*

What have we most likely inherited from our parents more than anything else?

Poor choices and habits.

Which foods contain "stealth sugars" in them?

Ketchup, breads, salad dressings, and crackers.

Jot down some examples of dead and living foods in the chart below:

EXAMPLES OF DEAD FOODS	EXAMPLES OF LIVING FOODS
Candy, cakes, pies, cookies, desserts, ice cream, soda, frozen dinners, french fries, chips, chicken strips, hot dogs, sausage, bologna, salami, lunch meats, bacon, margarine, shortening, and most commercial peanut butters	Fruits and vegetables, whole grains, seeds, nuts, legumes, beans, organic coffee, and organic dark chocolate (in moderation)

BE IN THE KNOW

Studies show that obesity is fast becoming the leading cause of preventable death and that the tendency to be overweight or obese can settle in as early as eleven years of age.

 SPEAK UP: Let's Talk About It

WHAT TO DO

Discussion questions are meant to promote interaction with the material on a personal level. Ask people to share their responses if they feel comfortable.

What dead foods have taken up residence in your diet?

Answers will vary.

What living foods do you already eat regularly?

Answers will vary.

Why is it difficult to choose living foods over dead foods?

Answers will vary.

Given the Scripture verses shared by the Colberts on the DVD and provided at the beginning of this chapter, how is this pillar relevant to our faith?

Answers will vary.

Additional notes:

_____

_____

_____

BE IN THE KNOW

Containers made by Ziploc, Glad, Tupperware, and Rubbermaid are usually safe, being made of plastics that lack harmful substances and won't leach into landfills. Ask for your meat to be wrapped in butcher paper instead of the plastics many grocery stores use for meat packaging that's similar to Stretch-Tite, Freeze-Tite, and Reynolds Wrap. Don't ever store your food in foil, as acidic foods like tomatoes or citrus will break down the metal and draw harmful residues into the food. Finally, keep your refrigerator at a temperature lower than 40 degrees Farenheit, and never store leftover meats in the refrigerator for longer than three days—these are both common reasons for contracting food poisoning.

PUT IT ALL IN MOTION: Creating an Action Plan

WHAT TO DO

Review the thought starters provided here to help spark some creative ideas for this week's action plans. Then instruct the group to turn to the appendix (page 76 in the workbook and page 101 in the leader's guide) to write their action plans. Give them five minutes to complete their plans, and then ask each person to share theirs with the group.

THOUGHT STARTERS FOR YOUR ACTION PLAN

- ► How will you change the way you order at your favorite restaurant?
- ► What dead food can you drop from your diet this week?
- ► What living foods will you purchase at the grocery store this week?
- ► Consider purchasing a steamer as an alternative to frying or microwaving otherwise good and living foods.
- ► Start counting the number of times you chew each bite this week. Move toward the goal of twenty to thirty chews per bite.

 TAKE IT WITH YOU: Home Study, Action, and Prayer
(15 minutes)

WHAT TO DO

Take prayer requests from the group. Share the home study assignment listed below, and remind everyone to keep up with their action plans—they will give a report on how they did at the next meeting. To finish the meeting, ask someone to close in prayer.

List prayer requests for this week here. Remember to pray for one another this week.

_____

_____

_____

_____

Close in prayer.

Keep up with this week's action plan.

Home study assignment: Read Days 15–21 in *The Seven Pillars of Health* and answer the Questions for Deeper Understanding on the following pages.

 Questions for Deeper Understanding Days 15–21

DAY 15 — — — — — — — — — — — — —

As Dr. Colbert says, everything we put in our mouths has the potential to produce life or death. How has your perspective on choosing food changed?

> *Answers will vary.*

In what ways are you caught in the trap of the "standard American diet"?

> *Answers will vary.*

DAY 16 — — — — — — — — — — — — —

Which of these bad food traps listed below are operating in your life, keeping you from choosing living foods? Next to each one that applies, space has been given to express how that trap has caught you.

> *Answers will vary. Allow group members to share how these traps show up in their lives*

- Bad foods are a habit.
- Bad foods are convenient.
- Bad foods are a vicious cycle.

Food additives can make bad foods addictive.

Bad foods give comfort.

Fill in the blanks.

- ▶ Food is not at the root of obesity; _choices_ are.
- ▶ People often look to food for _comfort_ when the Holy Spirit is the real source of it.
- ▶ Gluttony is a _spiritual_ and emotional problem first, and a dietary problem second.

Which statement in the Agreement to Lose Weight on page 71 in _The Seven Pillars of Health_ represents the biggest challenge for you? Why is it difficult? How will you handle and overcome the challenge?

> _Answers will vary._

DAY 17 — — — — — — — — — — — — — —

Before reading this section, what perspective did you believe God had about food and your eating habits?

> _Answers will vary._

How has your perspective on God's view now changed?

> _Answers will vary._

What benefits are attached to a primarily vegetarian lifestyle?

> _Vegetarians live longer and may have lower incidences of heart disease and cancer. A diet of vegetables, grains, and water was shown to produce a healthier appearance and ten times greater wisdom both in Daniel and the three Hebrew children. (See Daniel 1:8–21.)._

DAY 18 — — — — — — — — — — — — — —

Explain some ways refined sugar wreaks havoc on the body.

> _It makes you fat, accelerates the aging process, impairs your immune system, is linked to behavioral disorders, leads to osteoporosis, aggravates yeast problems, leads to type 2 diabetes, elevates cholesterol, and is addictive._

Given all the negative effects sugar can have on our bodies, list some sugar-filled foods that regularly crop up in your diet that you will want to consider avoiding.

Answers will vary.

When reading labels and choosing foods to buy, which fats and oils do you want to limit or avoid? Circle the correct answer for each.

Hydrogenated or partially hydrogenated fats	Good	Limit	(Avoid)
Extra-virgin olive oil	(Good)	Limit	Avoid
Saturated fats	Good	(Limit)	Avoid
Monounsaturated fats	(Good)	Limit	Avoid
Canola oil	Good	(Limit)	Avoid
Trans fats	Good	Limit	(Avoid)
Coconut oil	Good	(Limit)	Avoid
Polyunsaturated fats	Good	(Limit)	Avoid

DAY 19

Based on the information Dr. Colbert has given, indicate whether these substances signal dead food or living food. Write "D" for dead and "L" for living in the corresponding box for each.

L Wheat germ	**L** Seeds	**D** White sugar
D Margarine	**L** Red and black beans	**D** Instant oatmeal

L Nuts	D Grits	L Old-fashioned oatmeal
L Fiber	D Crackers	D French fries
D White bread	L Extra-virgin olive oil	D Corn syrup
D Popcorn	D MSG	D Aspartame
L Blueberries	D Shortening	L Avocados

List the positive effects of keeping a diet high in fruit and vegetable servings.

> A diet high in fruit and vegetable servings lowers risk of heart disease and cancer, reduces blood pressure, lowers levels of bad cholesterol, and provides concentrated amounts of vitamins, minerals, phytonutrients, and antioxidants.

What is the benefit of organic fruits and vegetables?

> They have not been tainted with artificial pesticides or chemical fertilizers.

DAY 20

Why is irradiation so dangerous?

> The radiation level in irradiated foods is equivalent to 10– 70 million chest X-rays. Substantial evidence suggests it is unsafe and may cause cancers, mutations, and chromosomal damage.

How can you eat meat more safely?

> Choose organic, free-range, or grass-fed meats, and always look for the leanest cuts, such as chicken breast or turkey breast. Turkey is one of the best meats to eat. Limit red meat intake to four to six ounces once or twice a week.

What is the good news about chocolate?

> *It can be good for you! Taken in small amounts, dark choco-late has been linked to longer life, lower blood pressure, and improved cholesterol.*

Which dairy products are best? Why?

> *Organic, low-fat, or skim dairy are best, as well as goat milk and low-fat organic yogurt. Goat milk causes fewer allergies and sensitivities than cow's milk; organic skim milk has no saturated fat and is much lower in calories than regular milk.*

DAY 21 — — — — — — — — — — — —

Dinnertime should be a joyful, beneficial time. What do you do to promote a warm, loving, peaceful environment at mealtimes?

> *Answers will vary.*

As 1 Corinthians 6:12 says, "'Everything is permissible for me'—but not everything is beneficial. 'Everything is permissible for me'—but I will not be mastered by anything." How can you apply this to your eating habits and food choices?

> *Answers will vary.*

WEEK 4: Leading the Charge

Your Knowledge Bank for the Week

Give Them a Sneak Peek: Exercise

A body without exercise is similar to a stagnant pond that's dead to life—it breeds decay and disease. Movement is what refreshes the body, clears it of toxins, builds its strength, and increases its energy.

Keeping with the analogy of the stagnant pond, Dr. Colbert and Mary begin this DVD segment by emphasizing the need to "stir the waters" of our bodies with exercise. Even though one Bible verse says, "Bodily exercise profits a little" (1 Tim. 4:8, NKJV), they remind us that walking was a way of life in Bible times. Our bodies need regular aerobic and anaerobic exercise, as well as a good, solid stretching regimen, to recoup the benefits of longer life and lasting health. This week, we will learn how to make walking or other forms of exercise a way of life as well as fun.

In the readings for Days 22–28, Dr. Colbert gives greater detail on the difference between aerobic and anaerobic exercise as well as the benefits to be gained by working with weights and calisthenics. He teaches us how to avoid muscle pain, how to determine our target heart rates, and how to make exercise a more natural part of our daily lives. He also offers fun alternatives to traditional exercise, such as Christian yoga, Tai Chi, Pilates, and ballroom dancing, while stressing the maxim "The exercise we enjoy is the exercise we will do!"

Key Points at a Glance

► When our bodies get stagnant, they become breeding grounds for disease.

► Exercise refreshes our bodies, renews our energy, and provides us with strength.

► The benefits of exercise are numerous. Exercise improves the immune system, helps maintain normal blood pressure, conditions the heart, and prevents heart disease. It helps control blood sugar and improves lymphatic flow. It tones the muscles, improves digestion, slows the aging process, sustains mental health, and improves the memory. Done correctly, it even helps you sleep better!

► Walking is one of the safest and easiest forms of aerobic exercise.

- When walking, go slow enough so you can talk but fast enough so you can't sing.

- Never exercise along a busy highway where toxic fumes and automobile exhaust can put your health at risk.

- When beginning an exercise program, begin with a low-intensity activity and gradually increase your level.

- Do five minutes of warm-up stretches before exercising and five minutes of cooling down afterward.

- Weight training and calisthenics are part of a holistic approach to exercise. They help to build strong bones and muscles.

- When weight training, perform the repetitions slowly and with proper technique.

- Stretching promotes flexibility and can serve as a good warm-up prior to exercise.

- Yoga, when balanced with a Christian perspective, is a great health alternative to more traditional exercise. It combines low-impact exercise with stretching and breathing.

- Tai Chi, an alternative form of exercise that's great for older people or those suffering from arthritis, brings slow, smooth muscle movements to the recovery of muscle mass, strength, and flexibility.

- Pilates is another form of low-intensity exercise with stretching, like yoga. It helps reduce stress while increasing flexibility and muscle tone.

- Ballroom dancing is a fun way to exercise without feeling as if you are doing it. It's also a great way for couples to reconnect and spend time together.

- Be on the lookout for passive exercise opportunities, such as gardening, walking the dog, parking farther away from your destination, or taking the stairs instead of the elevator.

- The exercise we enjoy is the exercise we will do—find something you enjoy doing!

PILLAR 4: Exercise

And everyone who competes for the prize is temperate in all things. Now they do it to obtain a perishable crown, but we for an imperishable crown. Therefore I run thus: not with uncertainty. Thus I fight: not as one who beats the air. But I discipline my body and bring it into subjection, lest, when I have preached to others, I myself should become disqualified.

—1 Corinthians 9:25–27, nkjv

[A woman] girds herself with strength, and strengthens her arms.

—Proverbs 31:17, nkjv

But they that wait upon the Lord shall renew their strength; they shall mount up with wings as eagles; they shall run, and not be weary; and they shall walk, and not faint.

—Isaiah 40:31

 HOOK UP: Let's Get Started (45 minutes)

Welcome; open with prayer (5 minutes)

Health checkup: homework review (30 minutes)

Action plan progress report (10 minutes)

WHAT TO DO

Welcome everyone back to the group and open the time with a short prayer. Then review the homework questions from last week. Invite volunteers to share answers as they feel comfortable. After the homework review, ask each group member to remind everyone of their action plan from the previous week and share how they did in keeping up with it.

HEADS UP: Scaling the Fourth Pillar (60 minutes)

WHAT TO DO

Give the group five minutes to complete their self-assessment quiz. Review each question by asking for a show of hands on the answers.

1. Which best describes your current activity level?

    ☐ Very active

    ☐ Somewhat active

    ☐ Not at all active

2. Which phrase(s) best describe you?

    ☐ I most often feel energized and fit.

    ☐ I could be in better shape, but I'm not sure it's worth the effort.

    ☐ I most often feel sluggish and stagnant.

    ☐ I'm in the best shape of my life.

3. What is your willingness to begin an exercise routine?

    ☐ Very willing

    ☐ Open to the idea

    ☐ Not very willing

4. Which, if any, of the following do you do on a regular basis?

    ☐ Take the stairs instead of the elevator

    ☐ Take the elevator

    ☐ Try to find a parking space closest to the door

    ☐ Drive to the grocery store even though it's only a half-mile from home

5. I have tried (or am presently doing) the following:

    ☐ Joining a fitness club

    ☐ Walking on a daily basis

☐ Using exercise DVDs or videotapes

6. Which of the following in #5 have you stuck with?

☐ Joining a fitness club

☐ Walking on a daily basis

☐ Using exercise DVDs or videotapes

☐ None of the above

7. If you are not exercising on a regular basis, why?

☐ Don't have time; too busy

☐ Too tired

☐ Lost interest

 LISTEN UP: Learning From the Expert

WHAT TO DO

Before playing the DVD, share some "Sneak Peek" information from your Knowledge Bank with the group. Start the DVD, and tell the group to answer the DVD questions as they watch. After the video, ask for volunteers to answer each question.

What happens when we don't "stir the waters" of the body with exercise?

Our bodies become stagnant, like a pond, and begin to breed disease.

What does our lymphatic system do for us?

Our lymphatic system is the cellular garbage system for our bodies. It cleanses our bodies of toxins, debris, bacteria, viruses, and other microbes. But in order to propel our lymphatic system into action, we have to move our bodies.

Name at least three benefits of exercise.

Exercise helps prevent cancer and heart disease. It conditions the heart, decreases our stress levels, promotes weight loss, and helps decrease our appetite. It also helps prevent diabetes, and it lowers blood sugar levels in diabetics.

What made the critical difference between both sets of rats subjected to high levels of stress?

> *Exercise made the critical difference in keeping the second group of rats well and healthy.*

What are the three essential components of a good exercise routine?

> *Aerobic exercise, anaerobic exercise, and stretching.*

BE IN THE KNOW

Our lymphatic system is the cellular garbage collector for our entire body. However, it only makes its rounds when we contract our muscles. For the well-being of our bodies, we need to move!

 SPEAK UP: Let's Talk About It

WHAT TO DO

Discussion questions are meant to promote interaction with the material on a personal level. Ask people to share their responses if they feel comfortable.

What is the best news you heard on the DVD?

> *Answers will vary.*

What exercise programs or routines have you tried before?

> *Answers will vary.*

What caused you to stick with them or stop doing them?

> *Answers will vary.*

How motivated do you feel to try the exercise pillar as Dr. Colbert presented it?

> *Answers will vary.*

Given the Scripture verses shared by the Colberts on the DVD and provided at the beginning of this chapter, how is this pillar relevant to our faith?

> *Answers will vary.*

Additional notes:

_____

_____

_____

BE IN THE KNOW

Practice the following stretch to improve posture and flexibility:

While standing, place your arms straight down at your sides. Make a fist with your hands, and then twist your fists backward so that your palms face in front of you. Try to maintain this posture for twenty to thirty seconds while breathing slowly and deeply—you should quickly notice an improvement in your posture!

 PUT IT ALL IN MOTION: Creating an Action Plan

WHAT TO DO

Review the thought starters provided here to help spark some creative ideas for personalized action plans. Then instruct the group to turn to the appendix (page 76 in the workbook and page 101 in the leader's guide) to write their action plans. Give them five minutes to complete their plans, and then ask each person to share theirs with the group.

THOUGHT STARTERS FOR YOUR ACTION PLAN

► Purchase a pedometer or good walking shoes this week.

► Whom might you ask to be your exercise partner a few times per week? Remember, most people need accountability. Simply commit to an exercise program for three weeks, and it usually becomes a habit.

► Check with your local community center for dance or exercise classes that begin soon, and register for the next class that sounds fun and motivating.

► Rent or purchase a Pilates or Christian yoga DVD from the video store or library.

► Check into hiring a certified personal trainer to start a weight-training program.

 TAKE IT WITH YOU: Home Study, Action, and Prayer
(15 minutes)

WHAT TO DO

Take prayer requests from the group. Share the home study assignment that is listed below, and remind everyone to keep up with their action plans—they will give a report on how they did at the next meeting. To finish the meeting, ask someone to close in prayer.

List prayer requests for this week here. Remember to pray for one another this week.

_____

_____

_____

_____

Close in prayer.

Keep up with this week's action plan.

Home study assignment: Read Days 22–28 in *The Seven Pillars of Health* and answer the Questions for Deeper Understanding on the following pages.

 Questions for Deeper Understanding Days 22–28

DAY 22 — — — — — — — — — — — — —

How does "stirring the waters" apply to our lives with exercise?

> *Our bodies are mostly water. In order keep them alive and thriving, just like a freshly running stream, we need to move them around!*

Why is movement necessary for our survival?

> *If we don't move, bacteria and other wastes begin to infect our bodies and have no way of being purged. As a result, we begin "swimming around" in toxins that begin to adversely affect our health.*

Use the rating legend to place your answers on the scales below:

> ### RATING LEGEND
> 1 = very little exercise
> 2 = low-level activity occasionally
> 3 = aerobic activity two to three times per week
> 4 = aerobic activity four to five times per week
> 5 = aerobic activity every day of the week
> 6 = vigorous daily exercise

Place an X on the appropriate number to rate your current level of activity.

1	2	3	4	5	6

Answers will vary.

Place an X to indicate a realistic and reasonable goal for you to achieve during the next three months.

1	2	3	4	5	6

Answers will vary.

DAY 23 — — — — — — — — — — — —

How does exercise rest the heart?

> *Exercising regularly causes our resting heart rate to beat about sixty to seventy beats per minute, which is significantly less than an inactive person. Also, the heart is fed with oxygen between beats—the slower the heart rate, the more oxygen flows to the heart.*

Which of the exercise benefits are most important to you?

> *Answers will vary.*

What are the health effects of our lymphatic system, and how are these positive effects linked to exercise?

> *Our lymphatic system disposes of cellular waste. It is only activated through muscle contraction or exercise.*

DAY 24 — — — — — — — — — — — —

Recall a time when you were exercising regularly (even if the only time you can recall was in your childhood). What motivated you to do it?

> *Answers will vary.*

What would help exercise become a more realistic part of your life right now?

> *Answers will vary.*

What, if anything, is stopping you from doing it?

> *Answers will vary.*

DAY 25 ── ── ── ── ── ── ── ── ── ── ── ── ──

Using the formula Dr. Colbert provides on page 129 in *The Seven Pillars of Health*, calculate your target heart rate.

> *Answers will vary.*

Which of these aerobic exercises would you like to try in the coming months?

> *Answers will vary.*

- [ ] Brisk walking
- [ ] Cycling
- [ ] Rowing
- [ ] Elliptical machine or glider
- [ ] Aerobic dance routines
- [ ] Singles tennis
- [ ] Basketball
- [ ] Swimming
- [ ] Ballroom dancing
- [ ] Other: _____

Set a realistic exercise commitment for yourself, and realize that the exercise you enjoy will be the one you commit to long-term. Remember to start slow and gradually work up to an increased level of activity.

> *Answers will vary.*

How can you avoid or treat muscle soreness?

> *Be sure to warm up and cool down before and after exercising. Perform easy stretching afterward. Start exercising briefly at a low intensity, and gradually increase your exercise time and intensity. Avoid making sudden major changes. Do some low-impact aerobic exercise to increase blood flow to the affected muscle groups. Gently massage and stretch the affected areas. Wait it out.*

DAY 26 — — — — — — — — — — — —

How do weight training and calisthenics benefit the body?

> *They increase metabolism to help burn fat, improve posture, provide better joint support, reduce the risk of injury in everyday activities, reverse the loss of muscle tissue for reasons of aging, help prevent osteoporosis, and increase the levels of important hormones in the body.*

Match the phrase in the left column with the phrase in right column that makes an accurate statement.

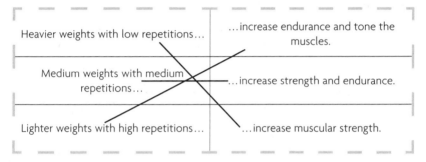

Heavier weights with low repetitions…	…increase endurance and tone the muscles.
Medium weights with medium repetitions…	…increase strength and endurance.
Lighter weights with high repetitions…	…increase muscular strength.

What kind of "fun" exercises, such as ballroom dancing or Pilates, have you tried before or want to try? What about it appeals to you?

> *Answers will vary.*

Visit www.bodyrecallinc.org or any other Web site that has to do with fitness. Make a note here of a few things you learned on the site that you can share at your next group meeting.

> *Answers will vary.*

DAY 28 — — — — — — — — — — — —

Take a few minutes to review Dr. Colbert's tips for exercise by filling in the blanks:

► Walk slowly enough so that you can _talk_ but fast enough so you can't _sing_.

► Never exercise near a busy highway where _fumes_ and _exhaust_ can put your health at risk.

► Do warm-up stretches for _five_ minutes before exercising and cool down for _three to five_ minutes after exercising.

- ▶ Drink plenty of water to replace what you are losing through sweat and _exhalation_.
- ▶ Never start exercising at _90_ percent of your heart rate.
- ▶ Don't exercise within _three_ hours of bedtime because it can cause insomnia.
- ▶ If life is stressing you out, add _exercise_ to your day.
- ▶ The best exercise for you is the one you _enjoy_.
- ▶ Schedule exercise as you would an important _appointment_.
- ▶ _Listen_ to your body.

Using the Activity and Calories Burned charts on pages 142–144 in _The Seven Pillars of Health_, estimate the answers to these questions.

- ▶ How many hours of playing golf with a golf cart would it take to burn off one Burger King Whopper?

  Almost four hours.

- ▶ When you eat that glazed doughnut at the office in the morning, how many hours of walking at 3 mph should you be prepared to do?

  One and one-half hours.

- ▶ What exercise might you engage in for one hour to burn off twenty Lays potato chips?

  Twenty minutes of brisk walking.

What dangers may affect those exercise enthusiasts who may be tempted to push their bodies too hard?

  Many suffer from chronic fatigue and muscle soreness.

WEEK 5: Leading The Charge

Your Knowledge Bank for the Week

Give Them a Sneak Peek: Detoxification

Whether we know it or not, toxins inhabit our bodies right now. They enter our bodies through what we eat, what we drink, the air we breathe, and the direct contact they have with our skin. That's why all of us need to implement the pillar of detoxification in our lives.

Dr. Colbert and Mary share that contaminants such as pesticides, chemicals, dust, smoke, and even heavy metals build up in our bodies in the course of everyday living, until the point of physical pain and other symptoms of ill health tell us our bodies have had enough. Even common substances, such as dental fillings made with mercury, can induce a type of "poisoning" into our systems. But the good news is, our bodies have a "waste management system" in place to clean up this kind of garbage. We can help it along by keeping outside toxins as minimally present in our lives as possible and by incorporating a few simple detoxification strategies in our lives.

In the readings for Days 29–35, Dr. Colbert informs us that toxic threats come from air pollution, indoor environments, food, heavy metals, and household and personal products. He explains how the liver and other bodily functions detoxify our systems and what we can do to help this process along. Key strategies include drinking pure water, eating chemical-free foods, and avoiding certain household products. The benefits of alkalizing foods and acidic foods, he says, are such that our bodies need a regular balance of both when we eat. We can easily start detoxifying our bodies through sweating, fasting, saunas, and "brushing" the skin.

Key Points at a Glance

- ▶ Toxicity permeates our environment. Our air, water, and food supply are filled with toxic levels of contaminants that increase annually.

- ▶ Mercury, found in most dental fillings, is one of the most toxic elements on the planet.

- ▶ Secondhand smoke is just as bad for you as cigarettes; breathing it for one hour has the same effect on your health as smoking four cigarettes.

- ▶ Organic foods are the only foods guaranteed to be free of pesticides and herbicides.

- In general, the thicker the peel, the safer the fruit.

- Pesticides and solvents, like household cleaning products, are fat soluble. Their chemicals get stored in the fatty tissues of our bodies, including the brain, breast, and prostate gland.

- Long-term exposure to dyes, insecticides, solvents, perfumes, and colognes may contribute to nerve damage and heart arrhythmias.

- Toxins may trigger most degenerative diseases, including cancer and heart disease.

- The "waste management system" in the body is designed to "take out the trash" on a daily basis.

- We need at least twenty-five to thirty grams of fiber each day to keep healthy.

- Perspiration rids the body of toxins—don't be afraid to sweat!

- Periodic fasting is one of the most powerful ways to detoxify our bodies.

PILLAR 5: Detoxification

My people are destroyed for lack of knowledge.

—HOSEA 4:6

And he that is to be cleansed shall wash his clothes, and shave off all his hair, and wash himself in water, that he may be clean.

—LEVITICUS 14:8

 HOOK UP: Let's Get Started (45 minutes)

Welcome; open with prayer (5 minutes)

Health checkup: homework review (30 minutes)

Action plan progress report (10 minutes)

> ### WHAT TO DO
>
> Welcome everyone back to the group and open the time with a short prayer. Then review the homework questions from last week. Invite volunteers to share answers as they feel comfortable. After the homework review, ask each group member to remind everyone of their action plan from the previous week and share how they did in keeping up with it.

 HEADS UP: Scaling the Fifth Pillar (60 minutes)

> ### WHAT TO DO
>
> Give the group five minutes to complete their self-assessment quiz. Then review each question by asking for a show of hands on each answer.

1. How often do you sweat?

   ☐ Daily

   ☐ Weekly

☐ Three or more times per week

☐ Never

2. How much time per week do you spend in the presence of someone who is smoking?

☐ No time

☐ One to two hours

☐ Two to five hours

☐ All my time

3. Do you ever have skin problems like strange breakouts, a rash, or itching?

☐ Yes, all the time

☐ Frequently enough to be a problem

☐ Occasionally

☐ Never

4. I eat organic foods:

☐ Exclusively

☐ When I can afford it

☐ Rarely

☐ Never

5. I have fillings in my teeth made of:

☐ Silver

☐ Gold

☐ Porcelain

☐ Composite

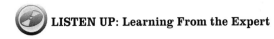 **LISTEN UP: Learning From the Expert**

WHAT TO DO

Before playing the DVD, share some "Sneak Peek" information from your Knowledge Bank with the group. Start the DVD, and tell the group to answer the DVD questions as they watch. After the video, ask for volunteers to answer each question.

What did the study of infant umbilical cords reveal?

The study found, on average, 287 contaminants in the blood of the umbilical cords, 180 of which were carcinogens. At least 217 of the contaminants found were toxic to the brain and nervous system.

What are the four greatest sources of pesticide exposure?

Air, food, water, and solvents.

When choosing non-organic produce, what rule of thumb will help you avoid pesticide exposure?

The thicker the peel, the safer the fruit.

Name a few simple keys Dr. Colbert gives for reducing pesticide exposure.

Decrease toxic exposure by drinking filtered water, eating organic food, and choosing leaner cuts of meat. Start breathing cleaner air by avoiding exhaust fumes, not exercising along busy streets, and staying away from secondhand smoke. Wear gloves when cleaning, and use natural alternatives to solvents.

BE IN THE KNOW

Cadmium—a natural element that's linked to lung damage, kidney disease, and high blood pressure—is one highly toxic chemical found in secondhand smoke, but that's not the only place we find it. Low levels of cadmium are found in many foods, especially shellfish and liver, and build up in the body over long periods of time. Those with diets low in calcium, iron, or protein are more prone to absorb higher levels of cadmium in their bodies.

SPEAK UP: Let's Talk About It

WHAT TO DO

Discussion questions are meant to promote interaction with the material on a personal level. Ask people to share their responses if they feel comfortable.

What surprised you about the information presented on the DVD?

> *Answers will vary.*

What hope was offered, despite such a difficult subject?

> *God has designed a powerful waste management team to help eliminate the toxins from our bodies. We can help this system perform more effectively by developing some key health habits.*

What questions did the video raise for you?

> *Answers will vary.*

Given the Scripture verses shared by the Colberts on the DVD and provided at the beginning of this chapter, how is this pillar relevant to our faith?

> *Answers will vary.*

Additional notes:

_____

_____

_____

BE IN THE KNOW

Exposure to pesticides—like those sprayed on fields where most of the produce in your local grocery store are raised—has been linked to the development of cancer, multiple sclerosis, epilepsy, and Parkinson's disease. There's no clearer way to say it—the sooner we go organic, the better!

PUT IT ALL IN MOTION: Creating an Action Plan

WHAT TO DO

Review the thought starters provided here to help spark some creative ideas for personalized action plans. Then instruct the group to turn to the appendix (page 76 in the workbook and page 101 in the leader's guide) to write their action plans. Give them five minutes to complete their plans, and then ask each person to share theirs with the group.

THOUGHT STARTERS FOR YOUR ACTION PLAN

- ► Take time for a sauna session.
- ► Wear gloves when you clean your house this week.
- ► Purchase pH strips to test your current urine pH level.
- ► Change your air conditioning filter. (This should be completed at least once a month.)
- ► Call your local waste management office to learn how to dispose of toxic chemicals in your garage or shed. Get rid of old paint, unused pesticides, and used automobile oil.
- ► Buy some green indoor plants or an air purifier for your home.
- ► Pick a day to complete a juice fast this week.

 TAKE IT WITH YOU: Home Study, Action, and Prayer
(15 minutes)

WHAT TO DO

Take prayer requests from the group. Share the home study assignment listed below, and remind everyone to keep up with their action plans—they will give a report on how they did at the next meeting. To finish the meeting, ask someone to close in prayer.

List prayer requests for this week here. Remember to pray for one another this week.

_____

_____

_____

_____

Close in prayer.

Keep up with this week's action plan.

Home study assignment: Read Days 29–35 in *The Seven Pillars of Health* and answer the Questions for Deeper Understanding on the following pages.

Questions for Deeper Understanding Days 29–35

DAY 29 — — — — — — — — — — — — —

How aware have you been of the need to detoxify?

Answers will vary.

What items in your home could be adding to the toxicity in your environment? Check all that apply.

Answers will vary.

- [ ] Old paint
- [ ] Old automobile oil
- [ ] Secondhand smoke
- [ ] Recently upholstered furniture
- [ ] New carpet or carpet cleaners
- [ ] Foods grown with pesticides
- [ ] Unused pesticides
- [ ] Dust
- [ ] Pet dander
- [ ] Spot removers
- [ ] Unsafe air deodorizers
- [ ] Chemical agents, such as ammonia, deep cleansers, furniture polish, etc.
- [ ] Other: _____

When was the last time you did something to help detoxify your body?

Answers will vary.

DAY 30 — — — — — — — — — — — — —

What indoor and outdoor toxins are you being exposed to in your daily life?

Answers will vary.

What foods do you normally eat that may be affected by pesticides?

Answers will vary.

DAY 31 — — — — — — — — — — — — —

Many common substances, such as dental fillings and vaccines, contain mercury or mercury-derived substances. How does mercury hurt our bodies?

Once mercury enters the membranes of our cells, our immune systems may identify our cells as abnormal. When this happens, the immune system will form antibodies to attack and destroy those "abnormal" cells. These attacks, over a long period of time, can lead to autoimmune diseases such as rheumatoid arthritis, lupus, Hashimoto's thyroiditis, Graves' disease, multiple sclerosis, fatigue, and muscle aches and pains.

What are the safer alternatives to silver fillings?

Composites and porcelain fillings, but realize that composites are only temporary.

Visit www.safecosmetics.org to learn about the safety levels of your personal care products. The Skin Deep Report allows you to search by name brand and product type. List your findings in the space below.

Answers will vary.

DAY 32 — — — — — — — — — — — — —

What toxic effects are you able to recognize in your life already, given some of the information you have now gained?

Answers will vary.

How can pesticide exposure affect our sex hormones and organs?

Pesticides have been linked to lower sperm count in men and higher amounts of xenoestrogens in women. In a 1980 study,

> *pesticides were found to produce structural abnormalities in the sex organs and hormones of male turtles, producing turtles that were unable to reproduce and that were neither male nor female.*

DAY 33 — — — — — — — — — — — — —

What foods help the liver perform its detoxification function?

> *Wasabi, broccoli, cabbage, brussels sprouts, kale, cauliflower, and all green foods.*

Why is it so important to eat fiber?

> *Fiber keeps the colon moving toxins along and out of our bodies on a regular, daily basis.*

List which alkalizing and acidic foods you regularly consume.

> *Answers will vary.*

How might you balance your food intake to be 50 percent alkaline and 50 percent acidic?

> *Answers will vary.*

DAY 34 — — — — — — — — — — — — —

What activities cause you to regularly work up a sweat during the week?

> *Answers will vary.*

If you aren't sweating on a regular basis in your weekly schedule, what can you do to change this pattern and increase your body's ability to detoxify through your skin?

> *Answers will vary.*

DAY 35 — — — — — — — — — — — — —

Mark the X column for the ways you already combat toxicity and the P column for ways you plan to begin combatting it.

> *Answers will vary.*

    X   P I use natural products like vinegar and lemon juice
             for cleaning.

    X   P I exercise aerobically a few times per week.

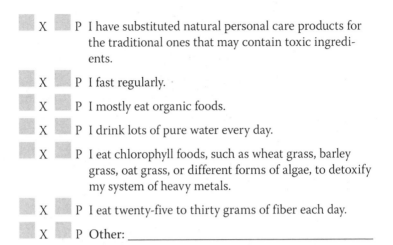

X P I have substituted natural personal care products for the traditional ones that may contain toxic ingredients.

X P I fast regularly.

X P I mostly eat organic foods.

X P I drink lots of pure water every day.

X P I eat chlorophyll foods, such as wheat grass, barley grass, oat grass, or different forms of algae, to detoxify my system of heavy metals.

X P I eat twenty-five to thirty grams of fiber each day.

X P Other: _____

Fill in the blanks below to review what you have learned about detoxification.

► Breathing *secondhand smoke* for one hour is the same as smoking four cigarettes.

► Staying well-*hydrated* with lots of water helps detoxify our bodies.

► Approximately 1 percent of our perspiration is usually *toxic waste*.

► *Alkaline* foods and water help raise the pH level of our tissues, enabling the body to release more toxins.

► Buy and eat *organic* foods whenever possible.

► Exchange your chemical-based cleaning products for natural products like *lemon juice* and *vinegar*.

► Replace your *air filter* every month.

► Eat twenty-five to thirty grams of *fiber* a day to support the health of your colon, the body's most important toxin disposal system.

WEEK 6: Leading the Charge

Your Knowledge Bank for the Week

Give Them a Sneak Peek: Nutritional Supplements

Few people get the nutrients they need from food alone. Some reasons are the depletion of nutrients in our soils, the over-processing that most foods endure, and the poor food choices we make on a daily basis, especially given all the choices available to us today. Because of these modern-day issues, Dr. Colbert insists that even the healthiest diet needs to be supplemented with vital nutrients.

This week Dr. Colbert and Mary discuss why a good diet isn't enough for good health. Given our environment and our behavior, we don't get the nutrients we need. Plus, each day we get hit with thousands of free radicals that set in motion an oxidation process of cell degeneration that is just not healthy for us. We need all the help that antioxidants, phytonutrients, and all the other essential vitamins can provide as we fight this battle for our bodies!

The readings for Days 36–42 give a closer look into the functions and benefits of each essential vitamin. Using helpful charts, Dr. Colbert explains what each vitamin does, what the daily dosage should be, and what happens when we don't get enough of it. He also warns against mega-dosing because of the harmful effects vitamins can have on our bodies if we have too much of them. Finally, Dr. Colbert dispels our "nutrition store phobia" by instructing us on exactly what kind of supplements and vitamins to purchase from those stores.

Key Points at a Glance

▶ Wholesome foods are the foundation of a healthy diet, but even the healthiest diet has to be supplemented with nutrients.

▶ An estimated 100 million Americans have digestive disorders. Even if they eat the right foods, their bodies may not adequately absorb the nutrients in the food because they lack the necessary enzymes.

▶ Antioxidants are to free radicals what water is to a raging forest fire. They protect us from diseases such as cancer and heart disease.

▶ Our bodies produce three key antioxidants—glutathione, superoxide dismutase (SOD), and catalase—that we need to sustain in adequate amounts. The five most important anti-oxidants are vitamin C, vitamin E, coenzyme Q_{10}, lipoic acid, and glutathione.

► A variety of fruits and vegetables provide us with a "rainbow of health" through the phytonutrients that give them their color. These foods also protect us from cancer and heart disease.

► Guidelines such as the recommended daily allowance (RDA) do not tell how much of a vitamin or nutrient you need to be healthy, but how much you need to prevent disease. Use it as a baseline goal for daily intake.

► When choosing a supplement, look for a whole-food multi-vitamin with 100 percent of the daily value of all thirteen vitamins and seventeen to twenty-two minerals. Also make sure you get omega-3 fats and phytonutrient powder in your daily supplement intake.

► Supplements do not replace a healthy diet; they complement it.

► Beware of supplements that contain toxic fillers.

► Taking supplements in high doses or excessive amounts can actually do more harm than good to our bodies.

PILLAR 6: Nutritional Supplements

God is not the author of confusion.

—1 CORINTHIANS 14:33

And he showed me a pure river of water of life, clear as crystal, proceeding from the throne of God and of the Lamb. In the middle of its street, and on either side of the river, was the tree of life, which bore twelve fruits, each tree yielding its fruit every month. The leaves of the tree were for the healing of the nations.

—REVELATION 22:1–2, NKJV

 HOOK UP: Let's Get Started (45 minutes)

Welcome; open with prayer (5 minutes)

Health checkup: homework review (30 minutes)

Action plan progress report (10 minutes)

WHAT TO DO

Welcome everyone back to the group and open the time with a short prayer. Then review the homework questions from last week. Invite volunteers to share answers as they feel comfortable. After the homework review, ask each group member to remind everyone of their action plan from the previous week and share how they did in keeping up with it.

 HEADS UP: Scaling the Sixth Pillar (60 minutes)

WHAT TO DO

Give the group five minutes to complete their self-assessment quiz. Review answers with a show of hands. Right answers have been provided for the questions that have them. Feel free to share the correct answers after asking volunteers to give their answers.

1. Which of the following supplements do you take on a daily basis?

   A multivitamin

   Ginkgo biloba

   Calcium

   Echinacea

   I don't take anything.

2. Which minerals can our bodies synthesize on their own?

   Iron and cobalt

   Chromium

   Potassium

   ✓ None

3. Which of the following best represents the average amount of a vitamin or mineral that is needed to meet the nutritional requirements of a person who is at least four years of age?

   Recommended daily allowance (RDA)

   Reference daily intake (RDI)

   ✓ Daily value (DV)

4. Proper digestion must take place in the:

   Mouth

   Stomach

   Small intestine

   ✓ All of the above

5. Everyone needs to supplement his or her diet with the following:

   A multivitamin

   A multivitamin and extra vitamin D

   ✓ A multivitamin, an omega-3 fish oil supplement, and a phytonutrient supplement

BE IN THE KNOW

Each cell in our bodies gets about ten thousand free-radical hits per day, and some researchers say we form millions of cancer cells each day. The only way to counteract this activity is with a regular intake of antioxidants and phytonutrients. Remember that an ounce of prevention is worth a pound of cure.

 LISTEN UP: Learning From the Expert

WHAT TO DO

Before playing the DVD, share some "Sneak Peek" information from your Knowledge Bank with the group. Start the DVD, and tell the group to answer the DVD questions as they watch. After the video, ask for volunteers to answer each question.

What was the shocking report put out by the *Journal of the American Medical Association* in 2002?

> *All adults should take a daily multivitamin supplement.*

What makes free radicals aggressive and therefore damaging to the body?

> *Since free radicals lack electrons, they attempt to grab electrons from surrounding cells, thus damaging the healthy cells and setting the stage for many cancers and degenerative diseases.*

What three antioxidants are produced naturally in our bodies through the intake of sufficient vitamins, minerals, fruits, and vegetables?

> *Superoxide dismutase (SOD), catalase, and glutathione.*

Why is lipoic acid considered the Michael Jordan of the antioxidant team?

> *Besides being a powerful detoxifier that protects the liver, lipoc acid also recycles the other four antioxidants and works in both fat-soluble and water-soluble components of the cells.*

What can we do to ensure we're getting all the phytonutrients we need?

Eat fruits and vegetables from every color of the rainbow.

BE IN THE KNOW

Isn't it interesting that God mandated a rest for the land every seven years? Leviticus 25:4 says, "But in the seventh year shall be a sabbath of rest unto the land, a sabbath for the LORD: thou shalt neither sow thy field, nor prune thy vineyard." The land needed to rest in order to recover valuable minerals.

 SPEAK UP: Let's Talk About It

WHAT TO DO

Discussion questions are meant to promote interaction with the material on a personal level. Ask people to share their responses if they feel comfortable.

What surprised you about the information in the video?

Answers will vary.

In what way have nutritional supplements been a part of your life before? If they haven't, why not?

Answers will vary.

In an area full of so many choices and complexities, we can start smart with what three basic supplements?

A whole-food multivitamin, an omega-3 fish oil supplement, and a phytonutrient supplement.

Given the Scripture verses shared by the Colberts on the DVD and provided at the beginning of this chapter, how is this pillar relevant to our faith?

Answers will vary.

Additional notes:

_____

_____

_____

BE IN THE KNOW

We need three to five thousand ORAC units per day to neutralize the free radicals produced in our bodies. ORAC units—nutritionist lingo for the antioxidant capacity in different foods—are most highly concentrated in Mexican red beans, wild blueberries, red kidney beans, cultivated blueberries, and cranberries. Clearly, berries and beans are our fiercest allies in the fight against free radicals!

 PUT IT ALL IN MOTION: Creating an Action Plan

WHAT TO DO

Review the thought starters provided here to help spark some creative ideas for personalized action plans. Then instruct the group to turn to the appendix (page 76 in the workbook and page 101 in the leader's guide) to write their action plans. Give them five minutes to complete their plans, and then ask each person to share theirs with the group.

THOUGHT STARTERS FOR YOUR ACTION PLAN

- ► Begin taking a whole-food multivitamin once a day.
- ► Purchase a week's supply of organic wild blueberries at your local health food store or grocery store.
- ► Increase your fruit and vegetable intake to the USDA-daily-recommended five to thirteen servings.
- ► Increase, decrease, or adjust the supplements you already take based on Dr. Colbert's advice.
- ► Schedule an appointment with your physician for a full "well man" or "well woman" exam.
- ► If you are over the age of fifty, purchase a supply of sublingual B_{12} tablets that you can begin taking daily.
- ► Instead of that morning espresso shot on your way to work, drink organic coffee or order a shot of wheat grass from your local smoothie shop. It will load you up with a burst of powerful antioxidants to neutralize many of those free radicals in your body.

TAKE IT WITH YOU: Home Study, Action, and Prayer
(15 minutes)

> ### WHAT TO DO
>
> Take prayer requests from the group. Share the home study assignment listed below, and remind everyone to keep up with their action plans—they will give a report on how they did at the next meeting. To finish the meeting, ask someone to close in prayer.

List prayer requests for this week here. Remember to pray for one another this week.

_____

_____

_____

_____

Close in prayer.

Keep up with this week's action plan.

Home study assignment: Read Days 36–42 in *The Seven Pillars of Health* and answer the Questions for Deeper Understanding on the following pages.

 Questions for Deeper Understanding Days 36–42

DAY 36 — — — — — — — — — — — — —

Why are multivitamins and supplements not just an alternative therapy but also a necessary part of everyone's daily nutrition?

> *We cannot get all the nutrients we need from our food, even if we have the healthiest of diets. Multivitamins and supplements ensure we get them on a daily basis.*

Fill in the blanks.

▶ Cooking and *improper food storage* strip away the nutrients from our food.

▶ Vegetables are most nutritious when eaten _steamed_ or _raw_.

▶ To be healthy, you need to start taking _nutritional supplements_.

▶ When we consume excessive amounts of liquids with meals, we wash out digestive _enzymes_.

Of the four ways of cooking vegetables—boiling, pressure cooking, microwaving, or steaming—which is the healthiest? Why?

> Steaming is the healthiest because it retains the highest percentage of nutrients.

What five things can we do to safeguard the enzymes in our diet?

> Avoid highly processed foods; chew food thoroughly; eat plenty of fruits, vegetables, and whole grains; avoid drinking excessive amounts of fluid with meals; and steam vegetables rather than cook them to death.

DAY 37

Why aren't vitamins considered "pep pills," as many people think they are?

> Vitamins are not meant to give instant energy but to assist with many biological processes, such as growth, digestion, mental alertness, and resistance to infection.

Complete the following tables for each vitamin and mineral.

VITAMIN E		
How it benefits my body:	**Sources I usually consume** *(circle all that apply):*	**What can happen if I'm deficient in it:**
Decreases free-radical damage; protects the heart, blood vessels, and breast tissue	Almonds Walnuts Macadamia nuts Cashews Eggs Oatmeal or oats (cooked) Wheat germ or wheat germ oil Sesame, sunflower, safflower, canola, or walnut oils Avocados Butter (organic) Chicken breast (free-range) Beef (free-range, extra lean)	*Neurological complications, which can result in an unsteady gait, decreased coordination of voluntary muscles, muscle weakness, peripheral neuropathy, and diminished reflexes* *Infertility* *Menstrual problems* *Miscarriages* *Shortened red blood cell lifespan*
Am I getting it often enough? Yes No		

MAGNESIUM		
How it benefits my body:	**Sources I usually consume** *(circle all that apply):*	**What can happen if I'm deficient in it:**
Needed for protein, fatty acid, and bone formation; prevents muscle spasms, heart attacks, and heart disease; lowers blood pressure; eases asthma; prevents constipation	Spinach Almonds Cashews Legumes Halibut or salmon Black-eyed peas Sunflower seeds Whole grains (rye, millet, and barley) Raw, leafy green vegetables Fermented tofu	*Loss of appetite* *Nausea* *Fatigue* *Personality changes* *Coronary spasms* *Muscle weakness* *Muscle twitches* *Irregular heartbeat* *Leg cramps* *Insomnia* *Eye twitches* *Constipation* *Headaches*
Am I getting it often enough? Yes No		

CALCIUM		
How it benefits my body:	**Sources I usually consume** *(circle all that apply):*	**What can happen if I'm deficient in it:**
Regulates nerve function and muscle and heart contractions; builds strong bones; prevents osteoporosis; lowers blood pressure; prevents colorectal cancer	Yogurt (organic, lowfat, plain) Turnips Kale Milk (organic skim) Cheese (organic lowfat) Tofu Cottage cheese (organic lowfat) Spinach Almonds Blackstrap molasses Broccoli Figs Sesame seeds Soybeans	*Osteoporosis or osteopenia* *Loss of teeth* *Loss of height* *Leg cramps* *Muscle cramps* *Hemorrhage*
Am I getting it often enough? ☐ Yes ☐ No		

VITAMIN A		
How it benefits my body:	**Sources I usually consume** *(circle all that apply):*	**What can happen if I'm deficient in it:**
Prevents blindness; repairs skin; forms bones and teeth; protects against flu and infections of the kidney, bladder, lungs, and mucous membranes; helps prevent cancer and heart disease	Carrots Apricots Leafy green vegetables Garlic Kale Peaches Red peppers Sweet potatoes Cod liver oil	*Frequent colds* *Dry hair and skin* *Skin disorders* *Sinusitis* *Insomnia*
Am I getting it often enough? ☐ Yes ☐ No		

VITAMIN C		
How it benefits my body:	**Sources I usually consume** *(circle all that apply):*	**What can happen if I'm deficient in it:**
Forms collagen; maintains bone, cartilage, muscle, and blood vessels; aids in healing wounds; helps prevent plaque formation in arteries	Red bell peppers Papayas Oranges Broccoli Strawberries Cantaloupe Guava	Fatigue Weakness Nosebleeds Swollen gums Arterial plaque buildup
Am I getting it often enough? ▢ Yes ▢ No		

VITAMIN K		
How it benefits my body:	**Sources I usually consume** *(circle all that apply):*	**What can happen if I'm deficient in it:**
Aids in blood clotting; regulates cellular growth; mineralizes bones	Broccoli Cauliflower Brussels sprouts Spinach Beef Swiss chard Cabbage Dark green, leafy vegetables Turnip greens	Increased risk of osteoporosis Easy bruising and bleeding
Am I getting it often enough? ▢ Yes ▢ No		

DIETARY FIBER		
How it benefits my body:	**Sources I usually consume (circle all that apply):**	**What can happen if I'm deficient in it:**
Controls cholesterol and blood sugar; controls irritable bowel syndrome, constipation, and gastrointestinal disorders; binds toxins in the GI tract; prevents gallstones	Wheat bran Psyllium seeds and husks Sweet potatoes Brussels sprouts	*Constipation* *Bowel irregularities* *Hemorrhoids* *Diverticulosis and diverticulitis* *Colorectal cancer* *Irritable bowel syndrome* *Elevated cholesterol* *Toxin buildup* *Poor blood sugar control (in diabetics)*
Am I getting it often enough? ▢ Yes ▢ No		

VITAMIN B$_6$		
How it benefits my body:	**Sources I usually consume (circle all that apply):**	**What can happen if I'm deficient in it:**
Aids in protein and red blood cell metabolism; assists the nervous and immune systems; helps keep blood sugar levels in normal range; helps form serotonin	Potatoes Fish Poultry Brussels sprouts Collard greens Brown rice Sunflower seeds Walnuts Chestnuts	*Skin irritation* *Headaches* *Sore tongue* *Depression* *Confusion* *Elevated homocysteine (a toxic amino acid associated with heart disease)* *Anemia* *PMS*
Am I getting it often enough? ▢ Yes ▢ No		

VITAMIN D		
How it benefits my body:	**Sources I usually consume (circle all that apply):**	**What can happen if I'm deficient in it:**
Absorbs calcium and phosphorus; develops strong bones and teeth; protects against cancer; helps prevent prostate cancer; may help prevent breast cancer	Salmon Fortified milk Cod liver oil Egg yolks Fatty fish, such as salmon Exposure to the sun	Osteoporosis Hip fracture
Am I getting it often enough? ☐ Yes ☐ No		

POTASSIUM			
How it benefits my body:	**Sources I usually consume (circle all that apply):**		**What can happen if I'm deficient in it:**
Maintains fluid balance; plays a role in muscle contraction; transmission of nerve impulses; releases energy from food; regulates blood pressure, levels of acidity, and neuromuscular function	Fish Potatoes Avocados Figs Raisins Prunes Apricots Bananas Grapefruit Oranges	Dairy products (organic lowfat or skim) Whole grains Sweet potatoes Squash Mustard greens Brussels sprouts Cantaloupe Peas Beans	Irregular heartbeat High blood pressure Wheezing and asthma Weakness Nausea Loss of appetite Altered mental state such as nervousness or depression Dry skin Insomnia Fatigue
Am I getting it often enough? ☐ Yes ☐ No			

Using the charts you just completed, name which vitamins you need to increase in your diet and the foods you can add that will satisfy the need.

Answers will vary.

DAY 38 — — — — — — — — — — — — — —

What are free radicals, and why are they dangerous?

Free radicals are atoms that lack electrons. They are danger-ous because they cause oxidation in our bodies, damaging cells and setting the stage for degeneration and disease.

How do antioxidants assist in curbing the activity of free radicals?

They neutralize free radicals.

What foods give us solid sources of antioxidants?

Fresh fruits and vegetables, cooked fish, meats, whole grains, egg yolks, milk, oatmeal, nuts, legumes, and green tea.

DAY 39 — — — — — — — — — — — — — —

What are cruciferous vegetables? How do they help the body?

Cruciferous vegetables contain two components that take the shape of a cross (thereby giving them the name "crucif-erous"). They contain more phytonutrients with anticancer properties than any other family of vegetables.

What are some examples of cruciferous vegetables?

Broccoli, cabbage, brussels sprouts, cauliflower, bok choy, kale, collard greens, and mustard greens.

Apply the phytonutrient "rainbow of color" to your life. List which fruits and vegetables in each color band you normally eat already.

Red _____

Red/purple _____

Orange _____

Orange/yellow _____

Yellow/green _____

Green _____

White/green _____

What foods will you add to round out each color band?

> *Answers will vary.*

DAY 40 — — — — — — — — — — — — — —

Why won't you be in optimal health even if you get 100 percent of your recommended daily allowance (RDA) of nutrients?

> *The RDA isn't a list of the amounts of nutrients you need to be healthy but a list of nutrients you need to avoid disease.*

With so much information and so many choices available, not to mention disagreement among health professionals, what does Dr. Colbert say you can be doing to safeguard your health?

> *Research the supplements you purchase. Don't use supplements that have been mass-produced for a reduced rate because these often contain inferior qualities and amounts of the nutrients you need, and they are usually synthetic with potentially toxic fillers.*

DAY 41 — — — — — — — — — — — — — —

What does it mean to mega-dose on vitamins and supplements?

> *Mega-dosing on supplements means using them the way doctors use medication—to treat symptoms instead of causes. People who mega-dose are taking more supplements than they need and generally have side effects due to their mega-dosing.*

Why is mega-dosing dangerous?

> *Pills contain more than mere vitamins or minerals; they may also contain binding agents, fillers, gels and gelatins, toxic fats, and dyes that can cause poor digestion and allergies. Also, mega-dosing can produce problems unique to each vitamin and mineral.*

Have you ever overdosed on something—a food, beverage, or even over-activity? What were the results?

> *Answers will vary.*

Balance is important in all areas of life. What part of your life is taking more of your energy and attention than it properly should? What steps can you take to bring it back to its proper balance?

> *Answers will vary.*

DAY 42 — — — — — — — — — — — — —

What is the danger of taking supplements in synthetic form?

> *Synthetic supplements are man-made instead of God-made. Our bodies don't get the combination of nutrients that characterize living foods. Synthetic pills isolate nutrients in high dosages, but living foods never provide nutrients in isolation.*

Why does Dr. Colbert recommend omega-3 fats so highly?

> *They decrease inflammation and thus help treat and prevent cancer, heart disease, rheumatoid arthritis, psoriasis, migraine headaches, allergies, Alzheimer's disease, and even diabetes.*

Based on what you now know, what "rules of thumb" will you follow when selecting and taking vitamins and supplements?

> *Select a whole-food multivitamin, since it will provide the essential nutrients in combination form rather than isolation. Include omega-3 fats and a phytonutrient powder in your daily supplement intake.*

Are the substances below a friend or foe to our bodies? Explain why.

SUBSTANCE	CIRCLE ONE	WHY?
Enzymes	(Friend) or Foe	*Aids in digestion and food absorption*
Hydrochloric acid	(Friend) or Foe	*Aids in digestion*
MSG	Friend or (Foe)	*Food additive and flavor enhancer; also an excitotoxin and may cause memory loss*
Flavonoids	(Friend) or Foe	*Nutrient*
Soluble fiber	(Friend) or Foe	*Found in plant cell walls*
Carotenoids	(Friend) or Foe	*Nutrient*
Free radicals	Friend or (Foe)	*Damage cells, tissues, and organs, setting the stage for degenerative disease*
Antioxidants	(Friend) or Foe	*Nutrient*

WEEK 7: Leading the Charge

Your Knowledge Bank for the Week

Give Them a Sneak Peek: Coping With Stress

Stress is a natural reaction of the body that enables us to deal effectively with pressurized situations in short bursts. When stress persists and becomes a way of life, however, trouble brews—stress begins to wreak havoc on our bodies, mind, and spirit, causing any number of health and emotional problems.

In this week's DVD presentation, Dr. Colbert and Mary share their experiences with stress and the techniques they have used to manage it. Simply put, stress stems from two places: things we can control and things we can't. All of us face uncontrollable stress factors, such as inclement weather or traffic jams, but we also face stress we can do something about. Two of the most effective ways we can reprogram ourselves to better deal with stress are through renewing our minds with God's Word and practicing gratitude on a daily basis.

In the readings for Days 43–50, Dr. Colbert outlines some very practical ways of disentangling ourselves from the snares of stress in our lives. We can live more mindfully, reframe our negative thoughts more actively, practice thankfulness and gratitude more regularly, and forgive others and ourselves more freely. He also exhorts us to maintain an adequate "margin" for stress in our lives, since it's an inevitable—and sometimes even positive—part of human life.

Key Points at a Glance

- Stress falls into two categories—situations we can control and situations we can't control.

- If we don't learn to manage stress well, it eventually affects our physical and emotional health.

- Practice mindfulness by training yourself to let go of anything other than the present moment.

- Express gratitude regularly.

- Be thankful for what you presently have, and resist the temptation to compare yourself or your possessions with others.

- Through reframing, shift your focus away from your present point of view to a larger, more encompassing, and positive perspective.

- Learn to envision the positive effects that will result from a difficult situation.

- Instead of complaining or worrying about disappointments, setbacks, or trials, begin to view these situations as teachable moments.

- Forgiveness significantly decreases stress levels.

- Eliminate unnecessary stress by building adequate margin into your schedule and finances.

- Practice proper abdominal breathing to de-stress the mind and body.

- Don't take on more activities than you can reasonably handle—learn the art of saying no.

- Limit the time you spend with pessimistic people.

- The promises in God's Word are meant to diminish the stress in our lives.

PILLAR 7: Coping With Stress

Therefore do not worry about tomorrow, for tomorrow will worry about its own things. Sufficient for the day is its own trouble.

—MATTHEW 6:34, NKJV

Be anxious for nothing, but in everything by prayer and supplication, with thanksgiving, let your requests be made known to God; and the peace of God, which surpasses all understanding, will guard your hearts and minds through Christ Jesus.

—PHILIPPIANS 4:6–7, NKJV

[Cast] down imaginations, and every high thing that exalteth itself against the knowledge of God, and [bring] into captivity *every* thought to the obedience of Christ.

—2 CORINTHIANS 10:5, EMPHASIS ADDED

 HOOK UP: Let's Get Started (45 minutes)

Welcome; open with prayer (5 minutes)

Health checkup: homework review (30 minutes)

Action plan progress report (10 minutes)

WHAT TO DO

Welcome everyone back to the group and open the time with a short prayer. Then review the homework questions from last week. Invite volunteers to share answers as they feel comfortable. After the homework review, ask each group member to remind everyone of their action plan from the previous week and share how they did in keeping up with it.

HEADS UP: Scaling the Seventh Pillar (60 minutes)

> ### WHAT TO DO
> Give the group five minutes to complete their self-assessment quiz. Review answers with a show of hands.

1. What are the top three stressors for you?

   ☐ Job stress

   ☐ Financial stress

   ☐ Marital stress

   ☐ Family situations or crises

   ☐ Stress over global issues (politics, government)

   ☐ Illness

   ☐ Other: _____

2. How often do you consciously thank the Lord during the day?

   ☐ For the food at each meal

   ☐ Periodically throughout the day

   ☐ When I'm sitting in a church service

   ☐ Maybe once or twice a week

   ☐ Once or twice a month

3. How often do you have a belly laugh?

   ☐ Never

   ☐ One to three times a day

   ☐ Three to six times a day

   ☐ Six to nine times a day

   ☐ More than ten times a day

4. When was the last time you practiced forgiving yourself as well as someone who offended you?

    ▢ Yesterday

    ▢ Today

    ▢ Last month

    ▢ I rarely (or never) practice forgiveness.

BE IN THE KNOW

Stress releases a sudden surge of adrenaline and the extra strength and mental acuity we need to thrive in highly charged situations, making it therefore a healthy and motivating part of life. It's only when prolonged periods of stress take up residence in our lives that we begin to suffer and lose a sense of well-being in life. We need to stress less and stress smart!

 LISTEN UP: Learning From the Expert

WHAT TO DO

Before playing the DVD, share some "Sneak Peek" information from your Knowledge Bank with the group. Start the DVD, and tell the group to answer the DVD questions as they watch. After the video, ask for volunteers to answer each question.

How does Dr. Colbert define "mindfulness"?

> *Enjoying the present moment, or learning to pay attention to what is happening from moment to moment.*

What does Dr. Colbert mean by "reframing"?

> *Shifting your focus away from your present point of view to see another person or situation from a new perspective.*

Name nine stress-reducing habits Dr. Colbert encourages us to implement in our lives regularly.

> *Mindfulness, reframing, laughter and joy, forgiveness, margin, meditating on God's Word, proper breathing,*

learning to say no, and surrounding ourselves with
positive people.

How many belly laughs should you get per day?

At least ten a day.

BE IN THE KNOW

The Bible teaches us in 2 Corinthians 10:5 to take *every* thought captive to the obedience of Christ, not *some* thought. If any thought is contrary to God's Word, we are to cast it out and refuse to think on it or rehash it. However, you alone are the gatekeeper to cast these negative thoughts and beliefs out of your mind. Choose to meditate instead on things that are true, honest, just, pure, lovely, of good report, virtuous, and praise-worthy, just as Philippians 4:8 teaches.

 SPEAK UP: Let's Talk About It

WHAT TO DO

Discussion questions are meant to promote interaction with the material on a personal level. Ask people to share their responses if they feel comfortable.

What situations have added stress to your life lately?

Answers will vary.

In what situations do you find yourself practicing mindfulness most naturally?

Answers will vary.

What sorts of things give you a hearty laugh?

Answers will vary.

Given the Scripture verses shared by the Colberts on the DVD and provided at the beginning of this chapter, how is this pillar relevant to our faith?

Answers will vary.

Additional notes:

_____

_____

_____

 PUT IT ALL IN MOTION: Creating an Action Plan

WHAT TO DO

Review the thought starters provided here to help spark some creative ideas for personalized action plans. Then instruct the group to turn to the appendix (page 76 in the workbook and page 101 in the leader's guide) to write their action plans. Give them five minutes to complete their plans, and then ask each person to share theirs with the group.

THOUGHT STARTERS FOR YOUR ACTION PLAN

- ► Start each day by giving thanks and saying, "This is the day that the Lord has made. I will rejoice and be glad in it!"
- ► Share reasons to give thanks with someone close to you.
- ► Express your gratitude to at least one person each day this week for something they have done.
- ► Spend five minutes each day practicing deep breathing.
- ► Subscribe to a clean "Joke a Day" e-mail list online.
- ► If you aren't ready to formally forgive someone for something they have done, start yourself on the road toward forgiveness by writing a letter—*one that you don't intend to send*—that expresses your true feelings about the situation.
- ► Remove or organize clutter items from your workspace, bedroom, or other frequently used living areas.
- ► Allow yourself to be "in the moment" when driving, working, talking, and sharing time with people at work and at home this week.
- ► Spend one day doing activities that are purely enjoyable all day long.

TAKE IT WITH YOU: Home Study, Action, and Prayer
(15 minutes)

WHAT TO DO

Take prayer requests from the group. Share the home study assignment that is listed below, and remind everyone to keep up with their action plans—they will give a report on how they did at the next meeting, which will be the very last meeting and a day of celebration. To finish this week's meeting, ask someone to close in prayer.

List prayer requests for this week here. Remember to pray for one another this week.

_____

_____

_____

_____

Close in prayer.

Keep up with this week's action plan.

Home study assignment: Read Days 43–50 in *The Seven Pillars of Health* and answer the Questions for Deeper Understanding on the following pages.

Questions for Deeper Understanding Days 43–50

DAY 43 — — — — — — — — — — — — —

Make a list of all the factors causing stress in your life right now.

Answers will vary.

Break each of the factors in the above list into the appropriate category below.

Things I Can Control	Things I Can't Control
Answers will vary.	*Answers will vary.*

List ways you can go about managing the stressors that you listed as being within your control.

Answers will vary.

DAY 44 —————————————————

In what ways has your own life experience mirrored that of Dan's, the man in the story that Dr. Colbert shared at the beginning of today's reading?

Answers will vary.

What moments and activities in your life don't resemble much mindfulness at all right now? In other words, when do you find yourself operating mostly on "autopilot"?

Answers will vary.

How can you convert those activities into more mindful moments?

Answers will vary.

List at least ten things—whether material, relational, or experiential—that you can give thanks for right now.

Answers will vary.

DAY 45 — — — — — — — — — — — — —

Identify some core negative beliefs rooted inside of you that have been the result of past experiences.

Answers will vary.

Reframe each of those core beliefs in a more positive light.

Answers will vary.

How do stress and negative emotions affect your heart?

> *They create erratic, disordered heart rate variability patterns, which cause the heart to send chaotic messages to the brain. This, in turn, causes our system to get out of sync and stressed out.*

DAY 46 — — — — — — — — — — — — —

On a scale of 1 to 100, what percent of the time would you say you feel the following ways?

Answers will vary.

Happy: _____ percent of the time

Neutral: _____ percent of the time

Unhappy: _____ percent of the time

Why is laughter so good for us?

> *It lowers the stress hormones cortisol and epinephrine while increasing feel-good hormones. It keeps us living in the present moment and seeing things in a positive light.*

How can laughter help us?

> *It reduces stress, lowers blood pressure, reduces pain, elevates moods, boosts the immune system, improves brain functioning, protects the heart, connects us with others, fosters instant relaxation, and makes us feel good.*

DAY 47 — — — — — — — — — — — — —

What types of moments do you find yourself rehashing in your mind?

Answers will vary.

In what areas of life are you aware of the need to forgive others?

Answers will vary.

In what ways do you need to experience the power of self-forgiveness?

Answers will vary.

DAY 48 — — — — — — — — — — — — —

Why is margin considered the difference between vitality and exhaustion?

When we build margin into our schedule, we gain breathing room and store up reserve energy. If we operate without margin, we run ourselves ragged going from one thing that needs to be done to the next and adding significant stress to our lives.

Where do you see the need to incorporate room for more margin in your life?

Answers will vary.

How can you purposefully plan and create room for more margin?

Answers will vary.

DAY 49 — — — — — — — — — — — — —

What seemingly harmless factors may exist in your environment right now that might be causing passive forms of stress?

Answers may include loud music, soap operas, gossip shows, depressing lyrics, dramatic television shows, or an inability to say no to others' requests.

Why is meditating on the Bible the most important foundation for a stress-less life?

Because the Word of God is spirit and life (John 6:63) and because the Bible says in Isaiah 26:3, "Thou wilt keep him in perfect peace, whose mind is stayed on thee: because he trusteth in thee." The only way to peace and coping with stress is to exchange our stressful, anxious, and fearful thoughts with scriptures that speak about who we are in Christ Jesus.

DAY 50 — — — — — — — — — — — — — —

Congratulations! Today marks the fiftieth day of your commitment to live in divine health. What are the most powerful changes you have made in the past seven weeks that have changed your life?

Answers will vary.

What positive results have you already experienced?

Answers will vary.

Since the fiftieth year was considered the Year of Jubilee in the Hebrew calendar—a year when slaves were set free from their masters and debtors were released from all their debts—how do you feel that you have been set free and released from poor health, bad habits, and disease by participating in this program?

Answers will vary.

DAY 50: Your Day of Jubilee!

> Rejoice in the Lord alway: and again I say, Rejoice.
>
> —PHILIPPIANS 4:4

It's Day 50, which means you have completed your commitment to the seven-week study of *The Seven Pillars of Health*! This is cause for celebration, as well as reflection, on how life has changed in the past seven weeks.

WHAT TO DO

This last group meeting will run a bit differently than the others. There won't be a DVD to watch or homework to assign. There isn't any new information to learn. However, to help round out the study before moving into "celebration mode," you'll want to complete a review of last week's homework and follow up on the action plans each person made.

 HOOK UP: Let's Get Started (45 minutes)

Welcome; open with prayer (5 minutes)

Homework review (30 minutes)

Action plan progress report (10 minutes)

 SPEAK UP: Let's Talk About It (60 minutes)

WHAT TO DO

It's time to help your group members realize the concrete value this study has added to their lives. Lead them in considering the following questions. Don't feel obligated to cover every single question if time begins to run short.

What new patterns and habits have you adopted in the last seven weeks?

Answers will vary.

How has your physical health improved?

Answers will vary.

How has your emotional well-being been affected?

Answers will vary.

What parts of this study have been particularly significant for you?

Answers will vary.

What other steps toward health will you pursue from here?

Answers will vary.

 TAKE IT WITH YOU: Let's Celebrate! (15 minutes)

As a group, you've committed to one another and to health for seven weeks. Don't end things here. Go out and celebrate! Pick one of the following activities—or another one that your group chooses—to enjoy as a group within the next month. Be sure to get it on the calendar before this last meeting ends.

WHAT TO DO

As the leader, make sure your group decides on a fun activity to enjoy together, as well as a firm date to do it. Your group may have already discovered an affinity for certain types of activities in previous weeks that you can plan to do in place of the activities suggested here.

- ► Plan a hike for an upcoming Saturday—and remember to bring lots of water!

- ► Sign up for a local 5K run/walk race together. Consider collecting donations for your favorite health-related charity group.

- ▶ Introduce more people to *The Seven Pillars of Health* by starting new groups at your church, with each current group member leading or co-leading a new group.

- ▶ Schedule a potluck and game night. Invite each group member to bring his or her favorite healthy dish to share.

Now it's time to enjoy the fruit of your labor—you've earned it! And remember that these seven pillars of health, when practiced regularly, will not only add years to your life but new and vibrant life to your years.

APPENDIX

Action Plans

WEEK ONE

Action Plan for Pillar 1: Water

Date: _____/_____/_____

This week I commit to practicing the following behavior:

_____

_____

_____

WEEK TWO

Action Plan for Pillar 2: Sleep and Rest

Date: _____/_____/_____

This week I commit to practicing the following behavior:

_____

_____

_____

WEEK THREE

Action Plan for Pillar 3: Living Food

Date: ____/____/_____

This week I commit to practicing the following behavior:

_____

_____

_____

WEEK FOUR

Action Plan for Pillar 4: Exercise

Date: ____/____/_____

This week I commit to practicing the following behavior:

_____

_____

_____

WEEK FIVE

Action Plan for Pillar 5: Detoxification

Date: ____/____/_____

This week I commit to practicing the following behavior:

_____

_____

_____

WEEK SIX

Action Plan for Pillar 6: Nutritional Supplements

Date: _____/_____/_____

This week I commit to practicing the following behavior:

_____

_____

_____

WEEK SEVEN

Action Plan for Pillar 7: Coping With Stress

Date: _____/_____/_____

This week I commit to practicing the following behavior:

_____

_____

_____

NOTES

NOTES

NOTES

NOTES

NOTES

NOTES

NOTES